Introduction

This is a book about my experiences wi
suicidal behaviours as a teenager and y
want to read about such difficulties? As unpleasant or as miserable as that may seem I intend for this book to have multiple positive effects. But this all depends who you are and why you're reading it. You could be someone who knows very little about depression, self-harm or suicidal behaviours. I want this book to give you an insight as to what it's like for someone to experience real depression so that one day you can be better equipped to help someone through their struggles. You could be a parent, relative, friend or teacher of someone who's going through something similar to what I went through. I want this book to give you some kind of understanding of what that person could be thinking and feeling so you can support them into getting to a better place. Or, perhaps you're in a dark place yourself and you need answers, or, maybe you want to read something you can relate to? Either way, if you're going through similar mental and emotional struggles to me I *honestly* aim for this book to be of great value to you. I hope that my experiences with mental and emotional make you realise that you're not alone and that lots of people go through similar challenges. If you're someone who is fighting your own mental health battle I really want to inspire and motivate you into finding peace of mind and happiness. That may appear to something unachievable from your point of view and I can understand why. However it is not impossible. If I can do it so can you.

Each chapter is about a significant event in my life that had a real impact on me emotionally and mentally for different reasons. All of the events laid out in this book are completely true and is accurate to my past, with the exception that they may not be in the exact chronological order. After my struggles I tried to forget what I went through and move on but when I realised I could help people by sharing my experiences I suppose I had to dig them out of the old noggin once again. The funny thing is that the memories are so clear to me, I just can't put an exact date on them all. But for the purpose of this book I have put estimated dates.

I'm not going to hold back on any of the details of my past, especially my feelings. This is not for the reason of entertaining or shocking you; it's for the purpose of painting the clearest picture possible. If you're someone who wants to learn from my experiences for whatever reason then you will not learn if I'm vague will you? With that being said I must give the obligatory TRIGGER WARNING to those who are currently struggling, for those who are trying to recover or have had similar experiences. I don't want to upset or bring back horrific memories for anyone as that's not my intention but I know that certain things can associate with bad memories that can send your mind into places that you wish to stay away from.

But this book isn't all doom and gloom. I'm still here, otherwise this book would not be! I did overcome my problems and my goal, above all others, is to help others do the same. A lot went into getting peace of mind but for the purpose of keeping things simple I will share some key points as to how I overcame my struggles in the later chapters of this book. Whether you're trying to better yourself emotionally and mentally, or, whether you're intending on helping someone else do that then the lessons I learnt from overcoming self-harm, depression and suicidal behaviours will be of great value. Everyone goes through a different journey in but I'm confident you will able to take away something from this book and use it to benefit yourself or someone else, even if it's just a little inspiration to do better.

Anyway, you get the idea. But before you continue I will admit that whilst reading you will notice that I did some pretty selfish and stupid things. You may also be questioning why I felt the way that I did or wondering what the hell I was thinking. I ask that you don't judge me. I was a very different and immature person back then. I was young, naive and I had a very negative frame of mind. I'm not using this to cover myself but I want you to realise that people with this mind set do things that they would not have done otherwise. Depression, anxiety and other mental disorders play their part in influencing you into doing things that "normal" people would not understand. For those who don't suffer with a mental health problem I hope this books brings you to a better understanding and opens your mind a little bit more. There's already enough stigma around mental health and we all need to do our bit to make the rest of the world understand the cause and the effects better.

And, finally, I wish to say that when telling the story of my struggles it may appear that some of the closest people to me were not very nice to due to the way I have portrayed them. This includes my friends and family. I want you to understand that I loved them all dearly, even at times when I didn't get along with them, and I still do. They were going through this dark time along with me and they were learning as they went along, just as I was. They didn't know how to deal with me or my symptoms for a long time, but, they still loved me and wanted the best for me. I ask that you don't judge them either. They're great people and I wouldn't change them.

Chapter 1 – My Childhood

I was born and raised in Kent in June 1990. My Mum and Dad were both working parents but I got to spend enough time with them to develop a close relationship from an early age. I looked up to them both. My Dad got me into all sorts of cool geeky sci-fi and superhero related things and he used to sit down with me and play with me and my toys. He used to take me to boot fairs on the weekend and buy me Transformers toys to add to my collection. My mum was very affectionate and made me laugh a lot. I remember when she used to play Brit-pop songs, as these were all the rage in the mid-90s, and jump around to them with me. I spent more time with my mum as a young child because my dad worked more hours than she did. But this didn't mean that I favoured one parent over the other.

At the age of five my mum fell pregnant and eventually gave birth to my first brother. My brother, Joe, was born extremely prematurely and was in a hospital incubator for some time. "He's the size of an Action Man" everyone kept telling me. I hadn't seen him at this point so I imagined him to be very small and thin. When the day came when I could finally visit my little brother I was super excited, and a little confused too. I'd never had a sibling before and it was an unusual feeling to have as a five year old. Fortunately the lights in my light-up trainers had stopped working so that distracted me from the nervous and curious feelings I had.

I got to the hospital ward where he was being attended to nurses and I saw him lying there in a clear plastic box with tubes coming out of his mouth. It was an unusual thing for a five year old to look at.

I didn't know how to feel about the whole thing and I missed my mum being away from home. She wasn't at home as much as she was continuously watching over my new brother but I wanted my mum all to myself. I'd been looked after by my grandparents mostly whilst my brother was in care.

When Joe came home having him there wasn't so bad. Although I did feel a little left out. Having less attention took getting used to. I played with my toys on my own more often when he came home.
As time went on I became more accepting of this whole sibling thing and it became more enjoyable when my brother reached his first birthday. On his first birthday we had friends of the family round and their children, who were about my age and we played well together. As I was the oldest I did take advantage of the situation. In my room we played a game similar to pass the parcel and I was the one with the controls to the cassette stereo. We passed a box around the room between about five of us and in the box I had drawn a pretend poop cut it into shape. This sounds ridiculous I know but at the time it was highly amusing for a six year old. I stopped the music purposely so that one of my friends would open the box and find the pretend poop inside for the rest of us to laugh in his "misfortune". It was kind of cruel in hindsight.

At the age of seven, about a month or so before my eight birthday, my mum came to me and sat me down whilst we were alone. "Scott, I need to tell you something," she said with a very nervous voice, "I want to move house but your dad doesn't want to." She then went on to explain that she, my brother and I would move to another house and that my dad would be staying in our current house. Anyone reading this would instantly understand what this really means; my parents we getting a divorce. Being only seven years old I took what my mum said as gospel truth. In my little innocent child head it made sense. I had only known that mummies and daddies love each other and stay together forever. I'd never heard of parents breaking up. Because of this it didn't affect me hardly at all, not at the time anyway. In my head my parents loved each other and they loved me. But this vision of my family living in separate houses yet still loving each other became less and less real as time went on.
Between the time my mum announced that we would be moving and my eight birthday I became more and more aware of things that I never took notice of before. Before, during and after we moved my mum and dad seemed to be constantly arguing or speaking to each other in ways that made me feel uncomfortable. I had never seen my parents get along so poorly before. Sure, I had seen them argue before but I didn't think much of it. Now it was becoming the norm and I just accepted it. When we did move my Dad helped out with the moving of the furniture. It was nice to

see my Dad getting involved but deep down I wished we could have just stayed together as a family.

Living away from my Dad was becoming more real as each day passed in my new house. Fortunately I accepted it pretty quickly and got used to our new living arrangements because I was focused on school, my friends, playing with my toys and the fact my eight birthday was just around the corner.

I couldn't help but notice the phone calls my Mum and Dad had which seemed to be daily. I got dragged into a few of them. "Talk to your father because I don't want to", my Mum once said in a frustrated voice. I remember hearing my Dad's voice on the other end of the phone sounding rather sad and desperate. He requested that I put my Mum back on but she refused. I tried to convince my Mum to speak to him but it was no good. These kinds of incidences made me realise that the move to another house was actually the end of the perfect family that I thought I had. My parents didn't love each other any more. For reasons I didn't know at the time my Mum despised my Dad and my Dad was trying hard to be on good terms with her. I hated feeling in the middle and I'm sure plenty of people reading this can relate. My little brother was too young to understand what was going on but I had become completely aware of the situation.

When the day of my eight birthday arrived I was so hyped for it. I had invited most of my junior school class round to go to the park for a big game of football and then a party at my house. It felt strange because it was the first birthday I had with my parents being split up. The fact my Dad came and stayed with us all day made it feel like we were a family again.

It was a lovely sunny day, the perfect whether for a game of football. I had just received the England goalkeeper away kit for my birthday and I couldn't wait to try it out. We all got onto the pitch at a local park and there was my friends, my cousin and my Dad all playing this really serious game of football. I loved being the goalkeeper because I had always enjoyed diving around and using my hands. I felt like a hero every time I stopped the ball from going in. Watching my Dad run around with us and getting involved put a big smile on my face. It took my mind off the fact my parents had broken up. Plus my parents probably agreed beforehand that they would not argue on such an important day for me. I'm glad they didn't argue otherwise the day probably would have been ruined.

Over the next few years there were some significant changes to my life. My Dad was in a new relationship, I started secondary school and I had a potential step dad on the scene. My Mum's new partner, Nigel, was really cool. He had a cool car, was into Star Wars and loved video games. Most importantly he made my Mum happy, something that I didn't get to see much of before. My Dad's new girlfriend was pretty cool too. I met her on the way to seeing the new, at the time, American adaption of the Godzilla movie. Meeting my Mum and Dad's new partners' was another new experience that felt unusual. To me they were just new grown-ups and that meant that I had to actively practice my good manners. I never thought about them being parental figures or being a serious part of my life and spending time with them day in and day out. Subsequently my Mum's partner Nigel moved in with us and my Dad's partner moved in with him. I got used to the idea of living with new people quickly because it felt like I had two families and all the grown-ups were happy, although, it was still apparent that my Mum was not on pleasant speaking terms with my Dad. I just tried to stay out of it.

Another few years later and my life had progressed further. I was in my teenage years and doing typical teenage things; hanging out with friends, not wanting to be at home much, trying to avoid all responsibilities and desperately wanting a girlfriend.
My Dad had gone through several relationships by this time, which annoyed me a lot because I told him that I was fed up of meeting them. I just wanted my Dad to settle down and get into a stable relationship like he had done after he and my Mum split up. Although that didn't end well either. My Dad was made redundant in my early to mid teens and he didn't take it too well at first. My little Brother and I used to stay at my Dad's place on Thursday nights and after school on Fridays, and on a couple of occasions I returned to his house to find him drunk. Not completely intoxicated but enough for him to be considered irresponsible. Being a teenager was hard enough, and my Dad wasn't in the best frame of mind either, and this wasn't an enjoyable experience to deal with. As pissed off as I was I couldn't tell my Mum. I was worried that I wouldn't be able to see my Dad any more. No matter how much I felt like he let me down from time to time I still wanted to spend time with him.

Life at home with my Mum, Brother and Nigel was pretty ordinary at this point. It felt like I had a proper family again. My Mum and Nigel were still

together and we lived as a family should live; enjoying weekends out, nice home cooked meals every day, family holidays and cosy Christmases.
Even though my Mum and Dad weren't together any more I was just as content as I was as a before they broke up. It was stable and I never worried that we were going to go our separate ways again.
At the age of fourteen Nigel told my Brother and I that he was going to ask our Mum to marry him, but first, he wanted our consent. It was nice to be respected in this way. Up till now he and I had had our typical teenager versus parent arguments and the whole, "That's so unfair!" thing.
I looked up to Nigel and he was my male role model but sometimes I felt that I didn't meet his expectations. He worked really hard all of his life and he wanted me to do the same but as a teenager I just wasn't that driven to succeed. I was more interested in finding a real relationship with a girl, hanging out with friends and trying to come across as "cool".
He kept trying to push me towards a career of my choosing but I found it difficult to make up my mind. I always wanted to do something artistic because I loved being creative and expressing myself.
Due to his and my Mum's expectations of me I was nervous about telling them that I didn't want to go to university even though I had, sort of, made up my mind that I wanted to design cars. To cut to the chase that pipe dream didn't last long. Even though Nigel and my Mum were supportive I felt like I had something to live up to and not knowing what I wanted to do with my life made me feel under pressure. I didn't want to be a failure and I didn't want to let them down. It was too much for me. Fortunately I still had plenty of opportunities to play video games and ride my BMX about my local town.

I finally got my first girlfriend at the age of fifteen and my first kiss with her was just as exciting as I'd imagined it to be. Being in a relationship made all the difference in my life back then. It kept me out of the house and I needed that. As the days went by I felt more stressed out at home due to the increasing amount of arguments I seemed to be having with my Mum and Nigel. I felt like Nigel had it in for me sometimes. Of course I made mistakes and I was lazy like most teenagers are but what he used to say to me felt condescending. I tried to defend myself and it didn't work. Things with my Dad were rocky too. He was still going in and out of relationships and I still wanted him to settle down with someone who had the potential to be my Step-Mother. Was that too much to ask for? He was so stubborn about little things, a kind of "My way or the highway" approach to our arguments. One time after school we came back to his apartment and we hand an argument on the way home, not that I remember what it was about, and I just waited outside once he went inside because I didn't want to be around him. There were plenty of occasions where I felt like my Dad wasn't who I wanted him to be. I knew he loved me but it wasn't demonstrated in the way that I expected or wanted. It had been years since he had done anything interesting with my brother and I. Going into town or around our Grandparent's house was as interesting as it got. I made the most of these things but I wanted my Dad to deliver something a bit more fun like my Mum and Nigel did.

In October 2005 my Mum and Nigel got married. Still to this day it was one of the happiest days of my life, not just theirs. Even though we had our disagreements and even though I felt under pressure at home this day of celebration made it all worthwhile. For a couple of days I forgot all the times I felt belittled, pressured and judged. I forgot the times where I felt like I came below their expectations. I forgot the times where I felt like a disappointment. Truly, I was very happy for them and for the first time in a while I felt like my future was going to work out.

Chapter 2 – First Signs of Depression

Up until the age of fifteen I didn't know much about depression or other mental illnesses. I had heard the term "Depression" and about these "Emo kids that cut themselves" but that's all I really had to go on. I'd felt sad and upset before but I had no idea what depression felt like.
But several months before my sixteenth birthday I started to emotionally dip from time to time and lose control of my rational thoughts. Negativity was creeping in and positive thoughts came to my consciousness less frequently. What the fuck was happening to me? Why was this happening to me all of a sudden? I didn't feel overly strong in my own mind and I didn't even try to resist these negative thoughts and feelings. It's as if I was welcoming them. I even started to question whether being alive was worth it any more. All these thoughts and feelings that I was now having seemed to be coming at me very suddenly and unexpectedly.
I had had enough of the bullying, I had enough of feeling under pressure at home and I had enough of feeling like I was a failure. These were the things that bothered me the most. They played on my mind more and more as the days went by. I kept on thinking about how easy it would be

to kill myself and put a stop to all the emotional pain that I felt tormented by.

Just before turning sixteen I had been in a relationship that I ended poorly, I wasn't getting on with my parents and I was about to go on study leave for my final exams. I knew I wanted to go to the local girls' school to attend their Sixth Form mostly because that's what most of my friends were doing. They kept me distracted from my unpleasant thoughts. When I went to school or out into town and faced all the name calling and provocation I felt alright. I had a great group of friends around me that supported me. But I didn't open up to them about negative feelings because they bought me so much joy and because they seemed strong I didn't want to appear weak. Plus I wasn't sure how to approach them about it, or anyone for that matter. Almost every day I was hanging out with one friend or another and they all helped me forgot my troubles without them even knowing I had any. But that didn't mean my problems were gone. It just meant that they were temporarily buried.

When we broke up for exams I went to a party with my friends at one of their houses. This was my first opportunity to get drunk and I was looking forward to the experience. I don't remember much that night except for the fact that one of my guy friends and I made out. I never saw that one coming, although, I had some bi-curious desires previously. I also tried my first puff on a cigarette at that party too. It was quite enjoyable, well, I was drunk at this point so everything was enjoyable.
The next morning didn't agree with me too well. I felt like I'd been run over and that I had food poisoning. I will say with pride that I didn't throw up, but I did keep running to the toilet thinking that I would.
In the days after the party my negative thoughts and feelings started to surface again and it wasn't post-party blues. A few more days passed and I felt like I was just about surviving with a fake smile to mask my feelings. I went into school to take exams wishing that I didn't have to and I came home wishing I didn't have to either. I wanted to be around my friends all the time to escape my feelings but I knew that wasn't realistic. Going to my dad's house felt like a chore, being at home made me feel like I was constantly treading on egg shells and going anywhere in public alone started to make me feel very anxious. I was used to being called "grunger", "weirdo" and "gay" by this time, they were common insults to alternatively dressed people like me, but each time an insult was thrown my way I felt a little weaker inside. My self-esteem and confidence wasn't

where it used to be and I had little motivation to be strong any more. Things just felt too tough. But to anyone looking at me from the outside would question what I had to worry about. I had a caring family, a nice house, my family had a good amount of income, I had plenty of friends and I could have anything I wanted pretty much. What reasonable excuse did I have to feel sorry for myself most would argue.

One evening I was with my Mum at our house. My Brother had gone to bed and my Nigel was out working late as usual. Back then I preferred being at home when he was at work, I felt a little less pressurised. My Mum and I were talking when things got a little heated. To be honest I can't remember exactly how it started, I think we were talking about my academic future, but I remember the emotions I started to feel from that conversation like it was yesterday. It was like I was a tank of gas that was continuously being pumped with more and more gas until I couldn't take any more. All of a sudden I couldn't take anything any more, especially this conversation.
With little thought I lashed out with, "It's no wonder I feel like killing myself!" The penny had dropped. The cat was out of the bag. The truth had surfaced. I had never said a thing like this to anyone in my entire life. My inner demons were no longer a secret. I sat down in shock of myself and waited for my Mum's response. There was silence for a few seconds and we stared into each other's eyes. I had no idea what she was thinking. Should I have said that? Did I really mean it? I did mean it, but I had no plans at that point. The idea of suicide just came into my mind from time to time.
My Mum started to have tears in her eyes before she could say anything and I started to feel pretty guilty about putting this on her. My Mum had always been good to me. She supported me and showed me the level of affection I'd expect from a good parent. I know she didn't have an easy childhood or even young adulthood so my outburst must have been pretty hurtful.
She asked me, whilst holding back tears, what was making me feel that way. I didn't know where to begin and a large part of me didn't even want to open up about it.
For a few seconds I thought about how to word it. I had never conveyed my feelings like this before and it was hard to rationalise and put them into words. As soon as the first word came out the rest came pouring out. I explained how I felt about being verbally abused regularly at school, how I couldn't make up my mind about what I wanted to do with my life and

how I felt about my relationship with my Dad, but I found it hard to talk about how I felt about Nigel. Without a doubt I loved my Step-Dad, I made that clear to her. I felt guilty for saying this, as he was the man she loved, but I had to explain how he made me feel. I put it across that he made me feel belittled, ashamed and even worthless at times thanks to his condescending remarks and with how pushy he could be.

My Mum asked me some questions about everything that I had said, I suppose she wanted to know everything that was thinking now. After being questioned for what felt like an hour she suggested I see someone professional; a therapist of some sort. I hesitantly agreed.
I felt a little relieved after talking about my darkest feelings with my Mum, it was like an emotional weight was lifted, but I was nervous about seeing a therapist. I had no idea what to expect except for what I had seen in movies and on television. I imagined myself to be lying on couch talking about my feelings whilst a trained professional took notes and asked me a thousand questions.
My Mum made it clear that she didn't want me on any medication. She said that they can have side effects that make the user worse off. I didn't know much about the medication that was available about this kind of thing either. I just had this image in my mind of being in a straitjacket whilst in a padded room, that's what scared me the most.

The evening finally came when I was due my first counselling session. I felt so nervous going up there. My Mum alone took me and assured me that it would be fine. She said to speak my mind and only talk about what I feel comfortable with.
It was dark and cold by the time we turned up to what looked like a large converted house. It was daunting. I approached the front door whilst shaking a little. My stomach felt like it was doing backflips. But once we got through the front door it looked more something between a library and a doctor's waiting room. Smart, medical and comfortable you could say.
We sat and waited for someone to call for me, it was only minutes I waited I believe but it felt like an hour. Whilst sitting there my mind was all over the place, I couldn't process anything clearly and I was trying to focus on what I wanted to say. It was important that I got the information across successfully otherwise the therapy would be of no use to me.
I couldn't sit still either. My legs and hands were constantly jolting and I was swaying back and forth a little on my chair; my anxiety was at a high.

Eventually I was called in and before I left my Mum gave me a cuddle, it was just what I needed. Before entering the room I took a deep breath to try and calm the nerves. The lady, I've forgotten her name, brought me into this small room with very dim little lighting. I sat in a comfy chair next a window where I could look over a part of Gillingham town. It wasn't like I imagined. I was kind of hoping to lay down on a sofa but I thought, "This chair will do".
The lady seemed very comforting and explained that I could say anything I wanted and that nothing said would leave this room. I needed to hear that because I had a feeling that everything I said was going to be passed on to my Mum, which wouldn't have helped me open up at all.

I didn't quite know how to begin at first but then the lady gently asked me to just talk about the first thing that came to mind. I went on to talk about my family, bullies and my lack of a future goal. Then I couldn't stop talking. I felt myself speaking with anger at times and lethargically at other times. The conversation got more serious when I told her I felt like killing myself sometimes. It felt so strange that I was opening up to a complete stranger and I was telling her more about me and what was on my mind more than to anyone I actually knew. It was even stranger in the fact that she had very little reaction to the things that I was saying. Not that long ago I was telling my Mum that I hated living and it made her burst into tears but this therapist basically had an expressionless face. Of course it's her job and she's expected to be like that. She asked me if I took my suicidal thoughts seriously. I told her that I didn't and that it was more a *feeling* of wanting to because of the things that were stressing me out. I continued to talk about my feelings, including coming to terms with my bisexuality and how I would open up to my family about it.
I felt like she was listening to everything I was saying and it felt good. It was nice to be able to open up fully and not feel like I was being judged. It was strange at first but opening up to a stranger was easier than I thought it would be. Not being emotionally involved with the person listening does make it easier to speak your mind.

If you, the reader, are struggling and you've not opened up to a therapist I suggest you make a start in doing so. The idea of talking with a stranger about your most personal feelings and thoughts for the first time is a daunting concept, however, it's easy once you start. I know how easy it is to bottle up and hide what's going on inside you from your loved and trusted ones but you can't hold it in forever. Pressure eventually builds

until you can't control it any longer and then it comes out in destructive and unpleasant ways. You know what I'm talking about right? When those feelings and thoughts keep circulating throughout you and then you impulsively lash out on someone or yourself? Talking to people makes all the difference. Even if talking about your problems doesn't stop you from being destructive it will at least *soften the blow*.
This is easy for me to say now but I wish I understood back then how much of a difference opening up to the right people made. It might have saved me some real hassle and maybe I could have avoided some negative feelings and experiences.
I was probably told this beforehand, as I had a tendency to not listen through a lack of caring, but it turned out my first counselling session was more of an assessment. The lady whom I spoke to was really nice and I wanted to talk to her again but I was told my next chat would involve being seen by one of her colleagues. I felt pissed off because this wasn't what I'd expected and it felt like a real effort to explain my "life story" in a short space of time. As relieving as it was opening up, it was exhausting.

Following my first counselling session I had the rest of my exams and my emotions and thoughts were all over the place. I was stressed to say the least but I hid it well. To everyone else I seemed calm and cool about it but really I felt like my life depended on it. I wanted to live up to my parents expectations, well, Nigel's mostly. I already felt shitty about the whole thing when I had an interview for Sixth Form, prior to my exam results, at one of the other local schools. The deputy head mistress was unreasonable in my interview. I came in to her office and made an honest but light-hearted comment, "I've waited ages for this moment." In return I received a very harsh, "I've been up since 6am and I don't appreciate comments like that! Not a good start is it?" I only meant that I was excited to be going there. Really I didn't care, I just wanted to keep my parents happy. I couldn't help but feel more anxious about my education; exams, revision and this monster whose school I could be attending after the summer holidays.

Chapter 3 – The First Time I Self-harmed

Up till now I felt like I was just living to please other people, yet I found myself disappointing them and I was disappointing myself along the way. The pressure was building and I couldn't take it any more. As I lived my life, not that it felt like a life, I went from one place to the next with the feelings of anxiety, disappointment and frustration, all of which made me feel depressed. I was coming to terms with the fact that I'm probably suffering with depression. I kept asking myself, "Am I depressed?" I had nothing to compare it to but I knew I didn't feel happy any more. I had this numb sensation all over me most of the time when I was feeling unhappy, which I never had when before when compared with general sadness. "This must be depression" I thought to myself.

My relationship with my Mum, Dad and Step-dad were still uncomfortable. You could argue and say, "Every teenager goes through this with their family" and I can't disagree with you. The only difference between me and a large group of average teenagers is that my family relationships plus exams, plus low self-esteem, plus being bullied plus being confused about my sexual orientation led to serious depression. I couldn't work out whether I was straight, gay or somewhere in between. At the time there was a lot of pressure around your sexual preferences. At my school you got called gay for just about anything by the twats that attended my school. I wanted to be straight because it was "normal" and probably would have been easier but I had feelings towards guys too. It didn't bother as much as some of the other things that brought me down but I just wanted to figure who I was in that sense. Fortunately I had the courage to tell one of my male friends whom, I had couple of experimental sexual encounters with, that I had confirmed that I was bi-sexual. It felt so good to say that to someone, because I hadn't really said it to myself before. I spent too much time worrying about what people would think, especially my friends. It wasn't long before I had the courage to tell the rest of my friends and they accepted me with opens arms. That surprised and delighted me.
I never really spoke of the bullying to anyone. I think it's because I didn't have a specific bully that picked on me. It was just random kids that hurled nasty comments at me or tried pushing me about. And I thought it was normal for kids to get bullied. I was at the conclusion that the world was mostly a cruel place so I just kept my feelings to myself and tried to deal with it. This was a big mistake.

During our final exams we had study leave, this was just an excuse to screw around trying to keep myself busy playing video games, riding my BMX and hanging out with friends. It was also an opportunity to feel under more pressure as I was around my Mum and Nigel more. "You've got to put the time in if you want good grades." "You won't have a good career if you don't put the effort in." "You must revise for a couple of hours every day if you want to do well." These were common phrases that came my way and I was sick of hearing them. I cared a little bit but the constant nagging put me off and seriously demotivated me.

One evening, throughout the exam period, I sat there in my room thinking about everything that was going on in my life. I thought to myself, "I've had enough of this shit!" The pressure, the constant disappointment, the resentment, the feeling of emptiness and anxiety was at boiling point. All sorts of unpleasant things were going through my mind; frustration, fear, anger, sadness and destruction. It was overwhelming and I couldn't take it any more. I just wanted my mind to shut up.
I recently heard of people cutting themselves as a way of coping with stress and sadness. That's when it dawned upon me that this could be a good idea to get rid of this unbearable tension. I thought about it for a while before acting on it. It was a scary thought, even more scary than my suicidal thoughts because this was something I could make happen right now. I had no idea what path it would take me down. Was it going to hurt like it does when I cut myself unintentionally? What if someone asks me about any cuts on my skin? Where should I cut myself? There was a lot of adrenaline flowing through me at this stage. I was shaking too. But after pondering the idea I made the decision to go ahead and try it because I hoped it would calm me down. I've always been pretty experimental and this seemed like a thing I could try. A stopped thinking about what the consequences might be and looked around for something sharp. I remembered that I had a draw full of stationary to the left of me. I opened it up and saw it; a pair of scissors. "That will do," I thought. I spread the scissors apart and put one of the blades to my outer left arm. My heart was beating so fast it almost hurt. "Should I do this?" I kept thinking. I couldn't think clearly for long. "Fuck it!" I said, and with that I quickly pulled the scissors across my skin.

Everything around me seemed to stop. I felt like I was surrounded by nothing but silence and that I was disconnected from reality. I could feel my heart beating quickly still, but, my mind was so clear and peaceful. The static and noise in my head had completely gone. I slowly looked down at my arm and saw a cut that wasn't very deep at all but it was enough to draw a little blood. I felt this relief that I had never felt before, in fact it was like nothing I had felt before.

Suddenly I started to reconnect with reality again. The adrenaline was wearing off and I only just began to realise what I had done to myself. I went to the bathroom and wiped the cut with a wet piece of toilet roll. As it didn't bleed to much it was easy to clean and the blood dried quickly. I then realised I had to put on a long sleeve top because I thought it would be obvious, no matter what I did, that the cut was new as my family had seen my bare arms throughout the evening. Plus with my recent confession of suicidal thoughts this would have just caused more problem for me.
I stayed in my room for a little longer before going down stairs. I didn't want to appear to be hiding from my parents, especially when I got accused of being unsociable a lot of the time.
Upon reflection the first thought that came to mind was, "That felt good." But then a little guilt and shame came along too. I had already pondered suicide and now I proved to myself that I was capable of actually hurting myself. I knew I had to hide this and tell absolutely no one, not even my best friends and certainly not my parents. I had only one counselling session at this point still and I hadn't gotten used to the idea of opening up to people I cared about. This "self-harm" was something I was going to try and deal with on my own.

When the cut had healed into a small scab I had the courage to have it out and test to see what people would say. This wasn't for attention, it was to make sure that no one suspected anything. That almost backfired immediately when the only person who noticed it was my Mum and she asked, "How did you get that?" I had to lie to her otherwise I'd end up having another therapy session sooner than I hoped for and probably make her cry again. I think it was mostly guilt that kept me from telling the truth. "I grazed it on a wall." This was the best I could come up with. She asked me again to make sure I was telling the truth so I repeated myself with a more sincere and firm voice. Lying to my Mum about this didn't feel good. I never found lying to be useful and it generally made me worse off in the long run, especially as I was bad at it. From then on I decided not do hurt myself intensionally again. I believed it was too much hassle to hide and I was afraid to try it again to be honest.

Over the next week or so I didn't feel like self-harming. I managed to get another girlfriend, I got to see my friends a lot more and Nigel worked a lot during study leave so I felt happier and more in control of my emotions. I think cutting myself steered me away from the depths of my depression because it shocked and scared me that much, in my view it was way beyond anything I thought I was comfortable with. It scared me so much that I tried really hard to be my old self again; a typical teenager who wants to be in love and spend time with friends. I was coming to the end of my exams and I just wanted to get them out of the way so I could enjoy an extended summer holiday doing the things that made me happy. I believed that if I tried my best and went in with a positive attitude I would do ok. Ok was good enough for me, whether it was good enough for my parents or not I no longer let that bother me. I was starting to believe that there was hope for me yet.

Chapter 4 – Starting Sixth Form with Suicide in Mind

Not long after my exams had finished and my sixteenth birthday my girlfriend and I broke up. "It's not you it's me," I was told. She sat there and cried whilst telling me this. I was more confused and disappointed at first but when I went home to my Mum I felt empty as I put my arms around her after telling her the news. I had just got over the hurdle of exams, but I was still waiting on results to find out whether I was going to get into Sixth Form or not. Not only that, my family and I were due to move from one side of the city to the other. This was just another nail in the coffin that made my blood boil. I didn't want to move, I hated change and this was a big fucking change. We were going to move somewhere that was beyond walking and cycling distance if I wanted to meet with friends or go into town. We were moving to a much nicer area but it was isolated from everything that kept me going. I thought about living with my Dad for a while but I concluded that I wouldn't be any better off. Seeing him made things worse more often than not.
Being dumped didn't affect me as much as I thought it would at the time of the break up but when I had time to take it in properly it knocked my self-esteem. Having that on top of all the other things that happened in the past plus moving away from everyone started to influence me to take suicidal thoughts more seriously. The idea of self-harm became more appealing again too. I still had no idea what I wanted to do with my life, which lead to feeling under pressure from my Mum and Nigel, I was still being bullied for my alternative fashion style and I was going to be "isolated" from my friends; whom I needed to distract me. These were the sorts of things that consumed my mind. My focus was on all of these undesirable things. It was like my consciousness was obsessed with

reminding me of things that made me feel like shit. I didn't want to open up about it either. I also felt too trapped and depressed to focus on anything that was positive about my life. "How am I going to travel anywhere?" "Am I going to get to see my friends outside of Sixth Form hours?" "When am I going to feel happy at home?" "Does anybody really want me alive?" I was asking myself these sorts of questions over and over just hoping for an answer. Most people in my situation would have been able to deal with the changes, or at least better than I did, but depression makes it very difficult to feel motivated and come up with solutions, alternatives and sensible coping mechanisms.

We moved house during the summer holidays between finishing secondary school and starting Sixth Form. The house was really nice and having my own room was a bonus. Part of me enjoyed the fact house was a lot larger and that I would get some much needed privacy but it still didn't make up for the distance that it created for me. It was difficult to keep my mind off the negatives.

Once everything had settled down and we had set the place up I asked my mum how I was going to get to Sixth Form and see my friends. "You'll get the bus mostly and sometimes we can give you a lift," I was told. Great, the bus, another thing I dreaded. I associated the bus with bullies due to some unpleasant experiences I had with the fellow morons from my school. I used to get on certain bus journeys apprehensively, expecting something to be thrown at me. Maybe it wouldn't be so bad now? It was hard to have positive expectations of anything when unpleasant past experiences were cemented in my mind.

It wasn't long before the change from the life I once knew got to me. I resorted to my phone and the internet to contact my friends, letting them know that I still existed. I had a fear that they would lose interest in me if we didn't keep in contact. I was already convinced that my last girlfriend left me because she knew I was moving away, I didn't want to lose my friends over the same thing.

I hated the turn my life had taken. There was more tension at home; it seemed like I was being moaned at for something new everyday and I felt lower than ever. I resorted to self-harm again. I felt like I had no choice but to hurt myself if I wanted to get some inner peace. I know it sounds crazy but believed that self-harm was the only thing I could do be in control of my emotions. Now that I had more privacy I had more opportunities to get the relief that I needed. This time I waited for everyone to fall asleep and then I could use my scissors, but this time I'd be a little more aggressive with them than I was the first time. I felt more anger whilst cutting this time round and it was *so* satisfying. I didn't realise back then that it was the endorphins that my brain had released that made me feel relieved. There was nothing like it. The emotional pain would disappear in an instant once my skin was penetrated. Like the first time it wasn't deep but I had to clean it and cover it up to avoid suspicion. I had a feeling my Mum and Nigel would go ballistic if the noticed and cuts on me. I got away with it last time but I didn't think I could get away with it again.

During the summer holidays my alternative style was that of the "Emo" look. I had always wanted to fit in to some form of group and I wanted to feel attractive. Typical teenager right? This style suited me because it was dark, wacky and slightly feminine. It was a shame that Emos gained a stereotype that they all self-harmed. I did look like an Emo at this point and I did self-harm but I didn't hurt myself to be a part of a trend. It was common for people with the Emo style to wear arm warmers or wristbands. I made use of this to cover up the new cuts I made in my new room. I still didn't want anyone to ask questions and arm warmers made it easy to hide. The problem was going to bed hoping that I didn't bleed into my bed linen.
The morning after my first cutting session in my new house felt like a fresh start. After a good sleep and taking anger out on myself I woke up feeling more in control, that's what I thought anyway. My left arm was a little sore from cutting it and it was uncomfortable unlike the first time I tried self-harm at my old house. Putting arm warmers over the scabs was uncomfortable too. The cotton threads pulled on the scabbing as I rolled them down my arm. I then wondered if putting an arm warmer on would actually stop my mum asking questions. She had seen one cut before, which clearly aroused her suspicions, and would a cover-up actually keep me away from interrogation? "I'll have to put on long sleeves," I thought. But then I realised it was an extremely hot day in July and that would look ridiculous. I became anxious pretty quickly about what would be the best option to hide my cuts.
I decided to go with arm warmers on both arms as I thought this was the least suspicious option.
I went downstairs to my parents with anxious thoughts running through my head. "Will they ask about why I've got arm warmers on?" I got myself ready to argue that it was a part of my fashion choice and to leave me

alone. I said good morning to everyone, I was usually the last one awake, hoping that they wouldn't ask anything. My hands started to go clammy and my heart rate increased. "Good morning," they responded, and, that was all. I got away with it, no questions asked. But how long could I keep hiding this from them or anyone else for that matter? I already had it in my head that I was probably going to self-harm again and commit suicide sometime soon. I wasn't proud of what I had done but it was something that I was beginning to rely one as a way of escaping from my problems.

The summer holidays dragged out for me. As each day passed I kept convincing myself that suicide was the right option for me. It wasn't even hard to convince myself because I had accepted that my life was going nowhere and that everyone else's lives would be unburdened if I died. I wasn't sure of when I was going to do it exactly or how I was going to carry it out, I just knew that it would be after I started Sixth Form. Part of my hoped that when I started Sixth Form that everything would get better. I wondered if being with friends and gaining qualifications could save me. I wasn't very optimistic about that though. I believed that it was more likely that it would end up being shit like everything else in my life. During the summer holidays I had plenty of time to wallow in my own self-pity and live through new experiences that ended up in my mental bank of "reasons to self-harm and feel like a piece of shit." On one occasion I managed to meet with my friends, and my recent ex-girlfriend oddly enough, in one of the local towns to where I previously lived. I rode my BMX whilst the others walked with me. As we were going from one town to the next two tough looking guys, perhaps a couple of years older than us, walk passed and said, "Excuse me bruv." We moved to one side as we didn't want any trouble and I don't think they did either until my ex quietly did an impression of what they had just said. My friends and I looked at her and told her to keep quiet. As we walked a little behind the two guys they kept looking back at us and we were convinced that they heard us.
I started to get really anxious now. My arm had healed since my last incident with self-harm so my arms were out and I was in a state of trying to feel confident about myself. It was a lot easier to do when surrounded by my closest friends. As we got to the next town half of our group, including my ex, went into a video game store whilst I and two other friends waited outside. The two lads, plus two more, came over to us and demanded that we waited there whilst two of them dragged the rest of my friends out of the store. I had to hide my anxiety so as to not show any

fear, I didn't want them to see that I was scared. After a minute or so one of the guys from the initial incident emerged from the store and grunted, with his lower-class tone, "Tell your girlfriend to be more respectful." I explained that she wasn't my girlfriend and he angrily responded, "I don't care!" Three of the four guys were quite tall and came across intimidating but the fourth guy was shorter than me. This short lad must have felt confident because of how big his mates were. He looked at me and said something along the lines of, "You fucking grungers!" Then he spat at me. I had some scum-bag's saliva hanging from my wrist and I was fucking fuming. I wanted to retaliate but I knew that would have got me in more shit.
Even though I just went through an intimidating experience I didn't feel too low afterwards. Having my friends by my side made all the difference in how I felt. I managed to laugh and joke about it afterwards and it didn't play over and over in my mind like things usually did. I had very little desire to hang out with my ex-girlfriend after that though.

My starting date for Sixth Form was getting nearer now and I was due to go to my secondary school to pick up my GCSE results. Even though I mostly didn't care I still had butterflies in my stomach. I guess this was due to wanting to die but still hoping Sixth Form would save me. When I got my exam results I couldn't believe my luck. I had achieved enough grades to get into Sixth Form and do the courses I initially chose. I didn't get any A grades but I got what I needed. I felt even better when I overheard some of the "hard" kids in my year sarcastically shout out, "Wow I got an E grade." I couldn't help but laugh to myself.
I called all of my close relatives and made them aware of my achievement. The congratulations and feedback I got from them all really boosted my confidence, this was the first time in a while I had lots of positive comments come my way. I was used to being questioned and moaned at. I proudly travelled round to the school where I was going to attend Sixth Form and show them my certificates so I could start there in a couple of weeks. I was more careful around what I said to the Deputy Head Mistress this time.

Over the next few days, with a week or so to go before starting my next level of education, I stayed indoors and isolated myself more than usual. The problem with free time and not doing anything with it when you're suffering from depression is that all you tend to do is think depressive thoughts. You go into a downward spiral that you can't get out of.

Negative thoughts that I had on previous occasions kept coming into my mind and I allowed myself to dwell in them. I still couldn't make up my mind about what I was going to do in the future and with Sixth Form closing in on me I felt under pressure again. What if I went through Sixth Form, gained some qualifications and then still had no idea what I wanted to do? I sold myself on the idea that a lack of a future career goal meant that I was a failure. My friends told me what they wanted to do and this didn't help. Part of me wanted to play in a band. I was heavily into my rock and metal music, which wasn't hard to tell judging by the way I dressed, and I was learning to play guitar. But that dream was killed off when my mum told me it's difficult to do and all the kids want to do it these days.
Not knowing what to do with my life was really brining me down, and, the fragile relationship I had with my Mum, Dad and Nigel didn't help. I tried to stay out of their way as much as possible; even that got me into trouble when I received lectures from Nigel about how I need to be more involved with out family. I found it very easy to self-harm because of all these worries and frustrations. I continued to use scissors because it didn't cut deeply into my skin and I had to put some effort into slashing to make my skin bleed, which helped with the stress. This was slowly becoming an addiction and part of me enjoyed it. Not because I enjoyed hurting myself or seeing blood but because it was such a relief to let go of the things that were eating me up inside.

It wasn't long before I got found out though. I had been a little careless with myself and my self-harm habit got me exposed. I had spent time during the summer holidays convincing my Mum that I was doing better and that I didn't need to be seen by any therapist but that was about to change. One morning I had my arm warmers on and my Mum strongly requested that I took them off because she found a patch of blood in my bed. I couldn't believe that I made that mistake. I tried to say that I had a small nosebleed, but I used that excuse before and I was never a great liar. I had to hold my breath whilst slowly removing my arm warmers because I knew how she would react and the aftermath of changes that would follow.
As expected, she started to cry and ask me a hundred questions. She wanted to understand why I would do this to myself and it was difficult to explain without giving away that I still wanted to end my life. My mum insisted that I would have to see a counsellor again. I went along with whatever she said to make my life as easy as possible. I went on to explain

the same things I had said to her the first time I opened up to her, only this time told her I didn't like how Isolated I felt from my friends and how trapped I felt.
After a long and uncomfortable conversation I stayed in my Mum's company for a little while to not arouse any more suspicion. If I went straight to my room after questioning she'd assume I would be self-harming again. I hated being questioned about my mental state, I didn't like talking about my feelings and problems with people who I cared about because it made me feel guilty and ashamed.
That evening, when in my room, I had a long think about my future. I came to the conclusion that I would definitely be committing suicide and that it would be around Christmas. It wasn't hard to reach this decision. Now that I had been exposed I had another thing to manage in my head and it wasn't easy to control. Self-harm was hard enough to deal with but hiding it from my family was going to be a real challenge. I had put myself in a vicious circle; self-harm to relieve pressure, but then cause more pressure by trying to avoid a body search and more questions.
This was all too much for me. I felt like I was progressively losing control over my own actions and my life entirely. I only felt satisfied when I formed a plan to attend Sixth Form, get a weekend job and try to lead a normal life until I would kill myself. I found comfort in knowing I could die when I wanted to.

The summer holidays were over and the day of starting Sixth Form had arrived. I had only started working a weekend job in a restaurant a few days before and I started to feel less of a child and more of an adult, despite feeling like an outcasted child at home. After being dropped off at the school by my Mum I quickly found my friends with a big sense of relief. I was anxious enough as it was, and depressed, so seeing all my friends again lifted a little weight. We had no idea how we would be organised into forms and classes, we hoped that we would end up in the same forms.
My anxiety was quickly forgotten when I looked around and noticed how many attractive girls there were in Sixth Form. "Maybe my last days won't be so bad?" I thought. There weren't any guys that I felt attracted to as all but two guys attended my previous school, I never had any feelings towards to guys at my school.
After lining up and entering the common room our head of Sixth Form introduced himself, as did the deputy, and they assigned us to our forms. I only took in half of what they were saying because I was distracted by the

fact there were some very beautiful ladies around me and that I couldn't wait to end my life. I was met with disappointment when I learned that I was in a form where there only person I knew was going to be a guy from my previous school whom I had no interest in, and he probably had no interest in me either. Luckily for him he knew some of the girls in our form.

We all got sent upstairs to find our form rooms and when we reached our form room I felt resentment. I questioned whether going to Sixth Form was the right option for me. But I knew I couldn't change my mind now as I had a plan to stick to. "I just need to see this out for a while and then it will be over," I said to myself.

We went in to the form room and our form tutor introduced herself and explained how Sixth Form worked. We were made to introduce ourselves to each other after that. This was another thing I hated doing; telling people about myself. Before it was my turn I imagined myself telling everyone that I was suffering with depression, self-harming and planning on ending my life. It was amusing to imagine that. When it became my turn I just gave some bullshit about what I was into and what I wanted to do with my life. It was definitely easier to lie and hide my feelings from people whom I had no emotional relationship with. They didn't care anyway.

Over the next few weeks I found myself slowly adapting to my new routine at Sixth Form. To be honest it was a struggle. Even though I was only studying three subjects and had plenty of lesson-free time slots it was weighing me down. The lessons were not too difficult but the work I had to produce at home to contribute towards my end of year grades was exhausting. I went to each lesson with regret and came away from each lesson with regret. I had only been there a month and the work load, mixed with depression and my rocky relationship my parents at home, influenced me to keep constantly thinking about self-harm and suicide. I remember spending half my lessons pretending to pay attention when I would really be visualising myself committing suicide and self-harming. I found it way too easy to be distracted by these types of thoughts. Every single little thing that upset or angered me pushed me into thinking about how I could hurt myself, and, this happened all the time. A tutor telling me I had to do better, my parents telling me I had to do better, my friends being distant, people taking the piss out of my appearance; these thing happened regularly and it hurt me so much. An emotionally stable person could deal with these experiences but I was on a downward spiral and I could never see myself dealing with these situations. Because I was depressed and lacking any level of self-confidence I just gave up and took an emotional beating.

A couple of months into Sixth Form now and I was self-harming almost daily; it was consuming me. I wore arm warmers every day regardless if I self-harmed the night before or not because I would be healing from the day before that and the scars that had healed were very visible. Every day I would wait for night time to come by because that was the guaranteed time when I knew I could hurt myself without interruption. The self-harm addiction became so bad that the only thing I really looked forward to was night time when everyone in my house was asleep so I could cut. Of course I cared about my friends and family and even some of my hobbies but they weren't obsessions like the self-harm had become.
One thing that I was good at was making friends and pleasing other people, unless it was my parents. Sixth Form was just about bearable because I had made plenty of friends, guys and girls alike. I didn't want be at Sixth Form but I had to go if I wanted to make everyone believe I enjoyed being alive, at least the vast majority of the other students took a liking to me. Being around attractive girls that actually wanted to talk to me boosted my social confidence too, whereas before I struggled to talk to girls that I was attracted to.

A few of us one evening went out bowling for a fellow student's birthday; the first time a girl had invited me to a birthday celebration so I gladly accepted. We walked to one of the neighbouring towns after a day of Sixth Form to go and eat at a local fast food restaurant. It was very busy and noisy in there, I could just about make out what my friends were saying. When we were almost finished I noticed that in the corner of my eye that there was a group of "chavy" looking lads staring at us, mostly me. I tried to ignore it and continue with my conversation. When I looked again one from their group was walking towards our table. I started to panic because I knew where this was going. He stood over me and aggressively asked what I had just said about him, which I did not. He was clearly looking for an excuse to beat the crap out of me just because I was dressed in an alternative style. This wasn't the first time I had been verbally abused or confronted for having hair that covered half my face, black skinny jeans (these were still only available for women at the time) and wearing black eyeliner; you get the picture. I told him that I had said nothing about him or his mates but he claimed that he heard me say something about them. I was starting to shake but with suicide coming my way at some point I thought I'd be cheeky with him. I said to him, "How could you hear what I said in this loud and busy restaurant from all the way over there?" I knew he wasn't very smart as smart people don't look for trouble. He paused for a second and then told me that I would be wearing my dessert if I said anything about him again. As he walked away my anxiety calmed a bit but my depressed feelings hit me hard. I felt so deflated as we were trying to have a nice evening and this moron was trying to ruin my night.

We got up, left and made our way to the bowling alley. There was six of us in total; three guys and three girls. As we walked to the bowling alley my anxiety heightened because I noticed they were following us. The worst part was I knew they were after me. That guy never said anything to the others in our group, only me. Probably because I looked like an easy target, which I was to be fair. We walked as quickly as we could without looking like we were trying to get away from them but by the time we got to the front of the bowling alley it was too late.

As I tried to walk forward to get in the bowling alley entrance I felt myself being pulled back by my bag strap. I turned around and the same guy from earlier had something to say to me. He said that we had to go to the car park and fight otherwise he would punch me in the face there and then. I looked over his shoulder and I knew he was a coward. He had three mates with him that were much bigger than he was and he wanted a reasonable cause to hit me, self-defence basically. I knew my two guy friends, Lewis and Mike, would have my back as they weren't exactly small or timid. I did my best to hide how scared I was and this was fairly easy to achieve because I didn't care about my own well-being so any outcome, even death, would have been okay with me. Plus I had been studying Ju-Jitsu for three years so I knew I could handle myself if I had to. In a careful and controlled tone I responded with, "I don't fight so you'll have to knock me out here." To my surprise he grunted, "No!" and repeated his ridiculous request. The tension was pretty high. I could feel my friends behind me waiting for a move, as was I, and I could feel the stare of the other three lads. I asked him what I had done wrong to deserve this and the best he could come up with was that I said something about him. I didn't bother saying anything else because I knew I'd end up going in circles. I didn't know what else to do so I just stood there waiting to be punched.

As the small lad went to open his mouth again I heard a shout from the bowling alley entrance. The manager of the bowling alley threatened the

four guys with the police and they quickly walked off. The little guy shouted, "We will be waiting here for you!"
As I walked into the bowling alley that final sentence he expressed got stuck in my mind. "Would he really wait around for two to three hours?" I asked myself. "He might and if he does I will get fucked up," I thought next." Then I thought, "Nah, he won't wait that long, will he?" Anxiety doesn't make things simple or allow you to make your mind up easily.
I didn't play a single game of bowling for the two odd hours we were there. I felt like shit. I sat on the side lines staring off in to the distance replaying the previous events in my head. I had this little piece of shit's face burned into my consciousness along with the thought that he might be waiting for me once I got out of this place. I wanted to go home but I didn't want to leave in case he and his friends were waiting for me. My friends comforted me as best as they could but I couldn't shake off my feelings of distress and frustration.
Eventually the time came when we had to leave. It was about half nine and we had been there for a few hours. I had spent the last hour calming myself down and trying to get into a more stable state but now that it was time to go home I started to get really anxious again. "Would they really be out there after all this time?" I wondered. I had no choice but to bite the bullet and find out. The bowling alley was on a second floor in a shopping centre so there was only one way out, as taking a fire escape wasn't really a suitable option. I approached the entrance slowly, poking my head around the door frame. My friends escorted me and kept motivating me to get me to leave. I walked out the front door and looked round hoping not to see their faces. I felt so anxious it was making me nauseas.
The shopping centre was deserted. I couldn't see them or anyone else. I wasn't quite relieved yet as they could have been waiting outside the main building. My Mum was due to meet me not far from the entrance but that still meant I had to walk past an area where they could be waiting. I paced to the back entrance of the shopping centre, praying that the path was clear to my Mum's car.
So far so good; the entrance was clear. I got outside and listened carefully, just in case they were waiting around the corner. My friends offered to wait with me until my Mum arrived. When her car pulled up moments later I started to breathe normally again.
On the journey home I decided to tell my mum what had happened, which was unusual for me because I was keen on keeping my thoughts and feelings to myself. When we got home I knew what I was going to do

once everyone was asleep. I just had to wait out an hour or so. This time I was more angry than depressed. I had self-harmed many times by this point and I usually felt depressed and frustrated when cutting myself but tonight was pure hatred. Hatred for this bully and hatred for my life. I never understood why, and please don't assume I'm into stereotyping or being judgemental as I know everyone is different, Chavs and your typical sports gear wearing youths like to abuse, attack and bully people who dressed in alternative style clothes such as Goths, Emos, Skaters and Grungers. I never intended to discriminate against people who looked and acted different to myself and it really angered me that someone would do it to me.
The more I pictured that short little twat the more it made my blood boil. It made me even angrier knowing that if he had been on his own he would have done fuck all to me. Even writing this paragraph is making me little angry.
I fantasised fighting with him on our own because I probably would have taught him a great lesson about messing with people whom you would assume to be weak. But I couldn't sit and think all night, that wouldn't make me feel better at all. Only my scissors were going to help me relieve the anger that was brewing inside of me. I didn't hold back or limit myself this time. I just went for it and I would deal with the bloody mess in the morning.

Chapter 5 – My First Cry for Help Suicide Attempt

Six months later a lot had happened to me, not a lot of good either, except I now had a baby sister that I actually felt proud of. But she or anyone else wasn't enough for me to want to stay alive. Things at home were constantly getting tenser. I had a lot of course work to keep on top of and my parents, meaning my Mum and Nigel as my Dad didn't seem to take an interest in my school work, were on top me to get it done to their expectations.
I had this assignment to draw some real life objects and I chose my BMX bike and a plant to draw. I thought something complex would impress them. I drew them out using colouring pencils but my heart just wasn't in it. The end results looked poor and like a small child had done them. I knew it and so did my Mum and Nigel. When I showed them what I had drawn they were very disappointed in me, which they made clear, and said that I would have to start over. I knew that I'd be ending my life soon

so perfection in my coursework was of no importance to me. I didn't want to do any work of any kind but I had to otherwise I'd end up spilling the beans about wanting to commit suicide. I did the pictures again but this time I put more effort across to please my folks and get them off my back.

I had a weekend job working in a restaurant. I really enjoyed earning money but I felt a little out of place with some of the people who worked there, especially one of the managers. At the time I felt like he had no respect for me, probably because I didn't meet his expectations either. He would make condescending remarks to me and never gave me any encouragement to do better in my job.
I preferred my job to Sixth form because I got treated more like an adult and I had no work to take home with me. Plus there was some really cool people there and I didn't feel judged for being myself. There was plenty of people working at the restaurant that I would usually assume to want to bully or verbally abuse me due to their nature, style and interests but it was really pleasing to make friends with them. They didn't laugh at my hair cut, eyeliner, skinny jeans or taste in music and I wasn't disapproving of their ways of life. I wanted all the people in the outside world to accept me like the team did in the restaurant that I worked for.

I started seeing a counsellor regularly at home. I can't remember her name but she had long dark blonde curly hair and was in her late thirties or possibly early forties. She first came to my house and was introduced to me by the lady whom I previously had my first and only session with. When my Mum told me my counselling sessions would continue, after finding out that I was self-harming, I hoped that the lady that I saw first would continue to see me so I didn't have to explain my life over again. Plus I felt like I connected with her and that was comforting to me.
We had our regular sessions in the dining room with the door closed and we would sit at opposite ends of the dining table. She would drink her coffee and listen to what I had to say. At first these sessions felt like they were very helpful, mostly because I got to unload my dark thoughts and feelings onto someone whom I had no emotional connection with but after a while they felt useless. I never told my family that though. I convinced them that they were really helpful so that they wouldn't suspect any suicidal behaviours. I didn't even tell this counsellor that I was planning on killing myself. Why would I? Although she had to be discreet about what we spoke about she had the right to inform my parents if I was planning a suicide attempt.

She gave me some coping methods like placing a rubber band on my wrist and pinging it against my skin when I got the urge to cut myself but that didn't work for me. I told her I would try it and I did once, but, I just wasn't as satisfying as actually hurting myself. We spoke about self-harm from time to time but we ended up talking about my childhood and current family situations mostly. I didn't understand why I had to keep talking about it at first until she told me that some of my feelings may have been bottled up from when my Mum and Dad split up. I didn't want to believe it at first because when I thought back to those years I never remembered being sad or down or anything like that. Maybe I was too young to have developed the feelings I currently had and instead they were stored unconsciously for eight years and now they were coming out in ways I couldn't control?
When my counsellor explained this to me it just gave me another reason to want to cut myself.
From that point on I only went along with the sessions to deceive my family. I had no intention of opening up as much as I did before. I was just biding my time.

I also had a short relationship with a girl, a boy and had "fooled around" in between. Being sixteen I was very sexually driven. I don't know if this was a product of a mental state that made me so sexually active or if it was hormones or the fact that my ego had risen to a new height, even though deep down I just wanted to be liked by everyone. Strangely enough one of the few things I had developed confidence in was talking to boys and girls in a flirting sense. My Emo look got me a lot of attention, mostly abusive attention, but guys and girls took a liking to me and it boosted my ego. I thought I was quite attractive, it was one of the few things that I was actually proud of. The whole Emo look was rising in popularity and prior to Sixth Form I had never fitted into any look, style or group.
I had made friends with quite a few girls in my year group, as well as some of the younger years. I dated one girl in my form for about a week until she left me, for reasons I'm still uncertain of. Quite ridiculous I know. At least I got a kiss out of her.
I eventually grew fond of another girl called Charlotte, which was a surprise to me because she was the first girl I connected with that was a really good friend and I, for once, wasn't trying to flirt with her, at least not intentionally. Like the girl I was seeing for a week I confessed my feelings to Charlotte but I wasn't expecting much as I knew she had been in a serious relationship for a while. Why did I tell her instead of keeping it

to myself? Well, unlike my feelings about depression, self-harm and suicide I felt like I couldn't keep this in. Perhaps I was hoping she'd want to be with me instead of her boyfriend and that could have prevented my suicidal feelings. It never went anywhere but we remained good friends and that was more than enough to satisfy me. I still wanted to be with someone though, anyone really. I wanted to end my life but I wanted some companionship, or at least a little fun, before I went.

Out of the blue in the middle of the day I received a text message from someone I had only seen but never really spoken to. I had always been observant and I always looked out for people with an alternative style to potentially make friends with. Having friends made life a little easier and making new friends was one of the few things I actually found exciting. The girl I had received a text message from I had seen about at school, I knew she was in one of the lower years and I knew she was likely to be similar to me in a sense of style, personality, etc. I assumed so anyway. I went on the fact that she wore a studded belt and a chequered sweat band on her wrist to make a guess that she was willing to befriend me and not lure me into some sort of social trap.
But the text message wasn't just about being my friend, in fact, I wasn't even sure how she got my number. I didn't question it because it was of a sensitive nature and it took me by surprise. I did wonder how serious she was being in this message because it's not the sort of thing people openly discuss and it isn't the sort of thing that people decide upon easily. The text message was about her confessing that she wanted to commit suicide with me. I replied to her and explained that I was up for it too. I told no one of this, for obvious reasons, but I felt like I was going to dangerous territory. Not only was this girl younger than me but we had exchanged messages about suicide, which started to feel wrong very quickly. But for the first time I was connecting with someone who shared my feelings about life. Not only did she self-harm but she wanted to die too, just like me. To be honest it excited me a little too. More than it should have. As much as it felt wrong it felt good having this connection with someone.

It was a little while before I actually met with this girl for the first time but by the time I did she had introduced me to one of her friends at the school, another girl named Charlotte. I was told that she wanted to join our little pact. I was okay with this because I didn't want to do it alone and I was afraid that someone would drop out. The more who joined the less

likely I would be on my own if anyone changed their minds at the last minute.
I could only communicate to them via text or talk to them outside of the school as it was forbidden for Sixth Form boys to speak with girls of the lower years. I tried to do this once before and was caught by the deputy headmistress. She demanded that I go to her office to discuss my "offence" at lunch time. I couldn't let that happen again, not now that the girls I was friends with were planning to commit suicide with me.
We met outside of the school a few times and texted regularly to discuss how low we were feeling and how we were going to do it. Originally I had it in my mind that I was going to jump off of our local shopping centre building as I knew it was high up and there were no fences around the top car park.

It wasn't long before the girl who first text me changed her mind about the whole suicide thing. I wasn't overly bothered because Charlotte and I were getting along really well. I started to develop feelings for her too. I'm not sure if it's because she wanted to commit suicide or because I found her attractive or she seemed pretty cool, maybe it was all of those things. I didn't tell her straight away because to me it felt wrong with her being two years younger than me for some reason. When I did tell her she said she felt the same way about me.
It wasn't long before we got into a relationship, one that I felt needed to be a secret. She was okay with this because of our decision to die together but also we felt people would judge us for our age difference. As much as two years didn't sound much we had already been judged for other things and we didn't want any more hassle. I didn't tell a single friend of mine, not even my closest friends.

Self-harm changed for me once I got into a relationship with Charlotte. Instead of being completely alone and isolated I found myself texting her back and forth whilst cutting myself. One night, once my family had gone to sleep, we were texting each other about how shitty we though life was and both decided to start self-harming. I pulled out my usual pair of scissors, which had dried blood from a few nights previous, and started to slice slowly at my left wrist. I felt numb but my heart was racing. I stopped every time Charlotte sent me a text because I wanted to know what was going on her end. She explained that she was using a razor blade, something I had not yet used, and was sitting in her bathroom doing the same as me. After sending my responses, describing my feelings and my

current situation, I continued to cut. I wasn't as angry as I used to be when cutting, I felt more apathetic about life and sorry for myself. My attention on myself quickly changed when she sent me a text saying that she had cut her wrist and the bleeding wouldn't stop. I started to panic and my heart went into overdrive. All I could do was tell her to wake her Mum up and wait for a reply. I hoped it wasn't as serious as I imagining. I was imagining her lying dead on her bathroom floor and I started to shake all over. I cut myself a little more to relieve some tension.
After waiting a while she replied saying that the blood had stopped flowing and I could breathe normally again. When it was over I was in a form of shock and disbelief. What had happened? Did I really just self-harm with someone? Well, through texting at least. This wasn't like before. Usually I would hide from the world and hurt myself but this time I let someone in to my darkest secret. I wasn't sure if I satisfied or disgusted with myself. With the tension dying down inside of me I had to clean up my wrist and get some sleep.

My life was spinning out of control. I become more and more distant from my family, I tried to stay in my room as much as possible to avoid any mental health related questions and general arguments or comments that made me feel shitty about myself. I found myself not hanging out with some of my closest friends and instead I would hang out with people who were also suffering with depression and self-harming. Misery loves company as they say. One of my friends, a guy whom I had grown close to in my last years of secondary school and Sixth Form, had started to self-harm. I was unsure if he had been doing it a long time but I noticed it in an art lesson. This was the second time a friend of mine had cut themselves. The first time was in secondary school and I didn't really know much about it at that point. It wasn't as common in the early/mid 2000s as it is today.
When I noticed my friend had self-harmed I was upset and shocked, so much that I said it out loud and a lot of people in the lesson heard me. I felt disappointed in myself for reacting that way because I know how personal self-harm is but it took me by surprise and I felt bad for him. Upon reflection later I kept thinking about suicide more and more and I knew the time had come to start taking action. I was thinking about all the reasons why I had to do it. Even though I had already decided upon it some time ago I still had to convince myself. Thinking about suicide is one thing but making a definite decision about it is another. But in a strange

way it was more thrilling than depressing. I let go of a lot of things that were bothering me because I had now set a deadline.
I gave myself about two weeks, which was enough time to write all my notes to my loved ones.

I wrote letters to my friends, family and the staff of the restaurant where I worked. I always had a lot to say about good people. I enjoyed studying people and their behaviours because it gave me an easy way to understand and adapt to them. In each letter I told everyone how grateful I was for having them in my life and I mentioned my favourite moments with them. I also said that some of my personal belongings would be theirs upon my death.
As I was writing out my notes a part of me didn't want this to happen. I didn't want to hurt my loved ones, not even my parents. As much as they frustrated me, all three of them, I still loved them and knew they were good people. But life was so challenging for me and that outweighed my love for them.
The next day I handed out my letters, in sealed envelopes that had a message on them not to open till the date of my suicide, hoping that they would not read them yet. Looking back I was naïve to think that this was a good idea. If I got an envelope from a depressed friend saying, "Open on whatever date" I would open it straight away. Surprisingly no one did, not straight away at least.
Several days later I received a call on my mobile from one of my friends, Lewis, whom I gave a letter. It was a few days before attempting to end my life and he had spoken with my other friends that had letters. Lewis asked me why I was doing this and stressed at me not to do this but I told him I wanted to carry this out and put an end to my struggles. It wasn't a nice phone call as I had not told a friend verbally that I wanted to die before.

When the day of my death date came I woke up with mixed emotions. Part of me was excited but my survival instincts felt like they were trying to tell me something else. I was shaky and trying to hold it all in. I was like a bomb waiting to explode. I got ready to go out and meet with some of my friends for the last time, including Charlotte. By now only her best friend new about us being together. The thing is that all my friends knew I was planning on ending it today but, on my poor judgement, I was deluded in thinking they would just let me get on with it. This wasn't the case.

I was dropped off in Rochester by my Mum, who as none the wiser as to what was going to happen to me today, and I was due to meet my friends at a bus stop. I waited about twenty minutes for them to arrive and in that time I was getting really anxious. My stomach started to feel sick and my mind was in overdrive. When my friends, and Charlotte, approached me, and before I could say hello, they told me that they wouldn't let me kill myself. I stayed a small distance from them and lead them into the next town where the shopping centre was. As we walked they tried to convince me not to go through with it but my mind was already made up. None of them ran towards me though. I think this was because they didn't believe that I would do it. Even though the walk through the towns was slow everything felt fast around me. It was like I was moving slowly but the world around me was at a lightning pace and I couldn't focus very well.
When we finally got to the shopping centre I walked, with my friends following me, to the place where I had planned to jump from. I started to slow down with my heart racing and my stomach feeling more nauseous than before. My nerves were getting the best of me but my determination kept me walking to the higher levels of the building. I got closer and closer to the spot and two of my guy friends, Richard and Mike, ran to me and grabbed me by the arms. I struggled with them a little and gently asked them to let go of me. When they refused I let my arms drop for a second to try and deceive them by then quickly pulling myself forward but they were quick to react. I kept trying to pull away from them and I asked them to let me see the edge of the building. They held my arms and let me, hoping that it would put me off probably. I looked over the edge down at the busy city centre road. Cars were driving in both directions and I had a quick mental flash of landing face first into the road. I pulled a little harder and practically begged them to let me do it. They refused and I tried to pull away with all my might then shouted, "Just let me do it!"

They wrestled me to the ground and laid on top of me so that I couldn't get out of their grasp. Charlotte and another girl, the one who originally wanted to die with me, went to find a security guard. The next thing I know my friends get off of me as a police officer approaches us. All I thought about was going to a room with padded walls and a strait jacket. The officer kindly asked us to go with him out of public view. We walked down some stairs inside the building to meet with another officer then he then got out his notepad and started asking me questions. He was very empathic with me, which was comforting because I thought police officers

were meant to be firm with people like me. The officer asked for my personal details and why I was doing what I was doing. I told him that I probably wasn't going to follow through with my intentions, hoping that I wouldn't end up in some kind of mental hospital.
Once the questioning had ended the officer offered to drop my friends and I back into Strood where I could get a lift from Nigel, who was shopping at the time. All of us climbed into the back of a police van, which I found amusing because onlookers probably thought we were being arrested. I sat in silence most of the journey with my hand holding onto Charlotte's. I was planning how to approach my parents about this experience and it was making me more anxious than I already was. I had a strong feeling that it would end up in arguments rather than cuddles and understanding.
As we pulled up to the supermarket I could see Nigel's car and my stomach dropped. I didn't want to get out because I was scared of what he would say and do. I knew it wasn't going to be good. I got out of the van and said goodbye to my friends. Nigel and my little brother Joe came out of the supermarket and started walking towards the family car. "This is the moment of truth," I thought nervously. He looked across the car park and saw me with a police van behind me and I all I could say was, "It's not what you think," hoping that he would be calm about all this. The police officer explained to Nigel what had happened and I started to feel miserable very quickly. Once their conversation was over I got in the car and the three of us drove home. I sat in silence the whole way home as I hadn't a clue as to what I should say. Should I justify or defend myself, or just take a verbal beating? I didn't know. I wanted to say a lot of things but I just couldn't get the words out I wished that I did throw myself off that roof instead of enduring this awkward silence. The journey home was about twenty minutes long but it felt like an hour.
We arrived home and I followed Nigel and Joe through the front door with my head hanging low. My Mum was home and I knew this was going to be another one of those conversations where I'd end up cutting myself once everyone went to bed. Joe was told to go and play in his room whilst my parents and I had a talk, which really meant that I would be listening whilst they spoke at me.
Before I could get a word in Nigel had already started to tell my Mum everything, from what he thought he knew at least. The way in which he conveyed my actions to my Mum didn't surprise me at all but it still disappointed me. He explained his version of the event with both fear and frustration to my Mum rather than empathising. I couldn't decide

whether to look my Mum in the eye or stare at my feet. I started to feel emotionally sick with the whole thing. What the fuck had I got myself into and why didn't I finish what I set out to do? I blamed myself for the failure of jumping and not my friends. After Nigel finished ranting he snapped and almost aggressively asked me, "Don't you give a shit how we feel?" I didn't even know how to respond. I tried to think of an honest and clever way to answer but I was lost for words. My lips were trembling with fear and self-pity. I tried to speak but no real words of meaning came out, more like quiet noises. I started to cry as did my Mum.
Our tears defused the situation a little, I think Nigel had let out any remaining anger and could begin to empathise, something that I didn't see very often where my emotions and mental health were concerned. The three of us cuddled like never before; it was what I needed from them this whole time, not shouting and accusations. From then on I had a little more courage to explain that I felt under pressure about school work and that I felt bullied for being me, I didn't have the courage to tell them that I felt like a black sheep of the family or that I had recently relived the events of my Mum and Dads divorce in my head over and over again. I definitely didn't tell them that I was going to hurt myself again and that I still wanted to die. Some thoughts just weren't meant to be shared with anyone that I loved.

I went back to Sixth Form on the Monday and tried to pretend like nothing had happened.

Chapter 6 – Second and Serious Suicide Attempt

May 2007, a few months after taking my first step towards what I thought was a real suicide attempt. I kept thinking about that event and how I could learn from it to make a better attempt next time. I decided that I wouldn't tell anyone or give any hints this time. The more I thought about my first try the more I realised that my survival instincts took over to prevent any harm being done. I wasn't going to let that happen again. I had enough of waking up feeling miserable on a daily basis. I was sick and tired of hurting myself regularly because of how I felt about my life. And I didn't want to put up with the bull shit and negativity that I faced too often.

Not much had changed since going to the roof of that shopping centre. I was still receiving slander for dressing the way that I did and for self-harming. One boy in the year above me at Sixth Form openly asked me in the common room, in front of all the others, why I cut myself. I didn't want to answer but I was tired of being asked the same stupid question by people who didn't understand so I just said something along the lines of, "It's how I cope with the shit in my life." He didn't have much to say to that.

I consistently got called gay and was laughed at whilst walking the streets of my local towns. I never let the bullies see how much their words got to me because I knew it would make it worse. I always put on a fake smile to let them think it wasn't hurting me. I wasn't prepared to change the way I looked just to avoid verbal abuse, I was comfortable with who I was.

My relationship with my Mum, Nigel and my Dad was as fragile as ever. We still had our arguments and I still disappointed them regularly.

I was still in a secret relationship with Charlotte though, at least I had that to keep me going for the time being. We used to meet up after the school day had finished and we would walk to Rochester and sit in this spot I found that was pretty isolated. We would sit, cuddle, talk and kiss for a couple of hours before going home. It was a thing of beauty in my mind, from time to time it even redirected my mind away from suicidal thoughts.

On one occasion after school we decided to sit on a grass patch at the end of the road where my Nan's house was located. The two of us sat and spoke of our day, our frustrations and how we would end our lives at some point. Just being there with her and talking brought comfort to me, the kind of comfort that could make the idea of suicide easier to comprehend.

After an hour or so of talking a group of younger boys from my old school, most of them only a couple of years younger than me, started walking past us. Just as they walked past us they laughed and taunted us with typical comments about being a "Grunger" and "Goth". I was getting more and more sick of people mocking me for dressing in an alternative style. At the time I was more angry than anything else but when I got home I couldn't let go of their comments. Usually I could let things slip my mind but because it ruined my time with Charlotte it brought me back down to a low mood. One that resulted in me using a razor blade on myself. Oh yes, I had begun to use a razor blade rather than a pair of

scissors or a knife now. I found that I could put less effort into cutting myself and get more painful results, thus, more satisfaction and relief.
The next day I decided to risk going to the same spot with Charlotte again after school but this time I was feeling more reckless than usual, maybe somewhat courageous too. We sat at the same spot, spoke about similar things and listened to some music on my phone. I didn't particularly want the group of boys from the previous day to come by again but if they did I was more mentally prepared for it. Guess what, they did come. The same boys walked past and said the same things as before.
But I wasn't going to stand for it. This was the first time in years that I was ready to make a defensive move rather than take whatever came my way. As they were mocking us, mostly me for my eyeliner and skinny jeans (as they hadn't gone mainstream for men at the time), I stood up and aggressively shouted, "What the fuck did you just say about me!?" towards one of the boys whom I recognised from a time in my old school where he mocked me for being a prefect. He and the others went quiet instantly. I was pretty shocked myself as I half expected a brawl to break out. I repeated myself with a firm tone and this lad stared at the ground and in fear told me he said nothing about me. As satisfying as it was to be in control of a bunch of bullies I attempted to be a diplomat and said the following in an honest and firm manner, "Now, I've not got a problem with any of you lot but for whatever reason you've got a problem with me, I've done nothing wrong and I don't get it. You should get to know people before you judge them." I had always wanted to get the narrow minded people of the world to be more accepting of people like myself and that was my chance to make a small difference. But it didn't work. They boy whom I scared said nothing but once the group of ten or so boys got about 100m away they started to taunt me again. I laughed at their cowardice.

When the next day of school ended I had a strong feeling those lads would come along again and I was ready for a fight. Quite out of character for me because I was used to avoiding fights where possible but on this occasion I had some fighting spirit flowing through me. In retrospect it was more aggression and stupidity that was really circulating around my heart and head. I wanted those boys to be there and I wanted them to attack me so I get what I thought was justice.
I brought my nunchuks into school that day and hid them in my bag, hoping that no one would notice. I didn't tell anyone that I had them on me and that I was potentially going to be defending myself against a

group of lads if I had to. I hadn't had a fight since winning a sparring completion two years previous when I was learning Ju-Jitsu and, even though I was prepared to get hurt, I wanted to improve my chances with a weapon that I knew I could use without killing anyone accidentally.
Charlotte, my friend Michael and I headed towards the infamous patch of grass near my Nan's house. Michael was a big guy who, even though he was suffering with depression, could handle himself if he needed. I felt like I needed him there because his presence had the potential to get those boys to leave us alone for good. I couldn't have been more wrong.
So we sat there, having our usual chats about music, school and the things we found funny when I saw the group of boys approaching. The anxiety started to kick in. I unzipped my bag and moved things around so I could grab my nunchuks at any given moment with ease. I'd practised drawing them and using them the night before so I could have the upper hand if things got messy.
In the distance I noticed they had someone new with them. A guy that I recognised from being in the year below me. He had a reputation for fighting, I had seen him fight before. He wasn't fast nor skilled but he was larger and heavier that I was. Not so much taller but fairly fat. My heart started pounding because I had a strong feeling I was going to have to strike him with my wooden nunchuks to defend myself and that would probably make things worse in the long run. In a flash I saw myself hiding away from the world out of fear that he would hunt me down if I used a weapon. I feared that I'd get stabbed or something along those lines. He got nearer to us three and walking next to him was the lad from the previous day that I had confronted. He didn't look so scared this time but he still stayed back from me. He pointed to me and said, "That's the one." I tried to swallow my saliva with the driest throat you could imagine. This large and angry looking bully walked over to me whilst I sat there waiting for a kick to the face. I had my bag to the side of me, slightly out of his view, and I had my left hand in there with a firm grip on my nunchuks. I waited for him to make the first move should I could claim self-defence should it get to that stage.
He told me to get up but I refused. I didn't want come across as a complete coward, even though I was shitting myself. He then told me that he would kick me in the face if I didn't get up, which made me change my mind. I had a shoulder bag with me and it was over my shoulder so when I got up I could subtilty continue to have my hand on my nunchuks. I rose up slowly, keeping a firm grip on the nunchuks, and waited for either a

beating or some more verbal abuse. I was surprised that no one had noticed my hand being in my bag this whole time.
The large guy warned me and told me not to fuck with any of his friends, I confidently told him I would not. As I continued to look him in the eye one of his little associates stood behind him and asked him the most cowardly question I've ever heard, "If I hit him," referring to me, "and he hits me back, will you knock him out for me?" I wanted to laugh so hard at this little shit but I knew that would only make my situation much worse and by now I was hoping it would just come to a conclusion. The little runt didn't make a move a move on me and this large chunky oaf turned to Michael and said, believe it or not, "You're a bit fat aren't you?" Again, I had to hold my laughter in at his hypocritical statement, he was larger in the face and stomach than Michael was. He then continued with his taunts by threatening Michael with, "Don't get involved otherwise I'll put you in the road." He then turned back to me with his face of intimidation. I looked him in the eye and I tried to hold a facial expression that told him I wasn't afraid, even though I was very afraid.
With my hand still stuffed in my bag he firmly told me to not look him in the eye unless I wanted to get knocked out. I didn't feel like getting beaten up so I quickly looked at my feet.
There was a moment of silence, and, to my relief, the big bully told his friends to follow him and continue on their way. As I felt my heart starting to slow down and I was able to catch my breath he mocked me one last time with a poor attempt of an insult, "I'll buy you some mascara next time." I didn't wear mascara, I wore eyeliner, but telling him that wouldn't help.
They walked away and my anxiety turned into depression almost instantly, with, a portion of frustration to accompany it. I felt so fucking shitty.

June, that same year, I turned seventeen. My birthday wasn't that special but the following night was a Friday and I had planned on having a party at my Dad's flat in Rochester. I invited my friends from Sixth Form, and of course, Charlotte, whom only Michael knew that I was dating. I wanted to get wasted and forget my troubles. My friends were the best thing for me but naively I believed alcohol would cheer me up.
Once Sixth Form was over for the week I went booze shopping with my Dad. We took the lot home and I got myself ready for my biggest and wildest party yet. My friends started showing up one by one and I was grateful that so many turned up to celebrate with me. My closest friends

Lewis and Richard, whom were more outgoing than I was, brought life to the party, as they could drink more than me, and I felt I had to up my game a little. I drank a little quicker, trying to keep up with them. I felt myself drunk within the first hour of this party starting but I wasn't the drunkest. A girl, Emma, was already pretty wasted and was being sick into my Dad's kitchen sink. My Dad's flat was small and only had three rooms; a bedroom, a bathroom and the living area, which was integrated with an open kitchen. As funny as it was seeing someone throwing up so early in the night we all tried to ignore it, except Lewis, a true gentleman who kept Emma company and gave her some support until she could stand up without vomiting again.
A few hours into the night there were a dozen of us that were pretty drunk. My dad was in the pub just two doors down and he popped in every now and then to check on us, mostly to laugh at my drunken state. My ex, the one that lasted a week, showed up with her friends that I knew. One of her friends was the other Charlotte, the older and non-depressed one that I confessed my feelings to previously. It didn't feel awkward as my ex was ok with me and we knew our relationship wasn't meaningful.
The night was already full of typical teenage stupidity and what not. Charlotte, my girlfriend, and I had still not told anyone about our relationship and that ended up being a detrimental factor. Not that it was his fault, as he was none the wiser, Lewis and Charlotte ending up having a drunken kiss. So did Richard and Charlotte, which backlashed as his girlfriend was at the party too. I didn't find this out till much later in the night when she was sitting and crying with Richard at the front door of the building. I don't know if it was the alcohol or my flexible teenage sexual desires that made it easy to accept that Charlotte had kissed two of my best friends. I told her I was okay with it, at the time at least. I used this as an excuse to try and make out with another girl whom I wasn't that close to.

Before midnight hit I couldn't drink any more, I was more drunk than I had ever been and I had lost complete control of my thoughts and feelings, so much so that I was overcome with my depressive feelings again. I had been having such a great night but out of nowhere I began to feel really low. Nothing triggered me as such, it was probably the alcohol that I couldn't handle, but I could feel my emotional high quickly dropping and fading into a pit of despair.

I sat in the corner of my Dad's flat with my mind replaying recent events; from the first suicide attempt to the problems at home and the bullying that I faced. With all the alcohol flowing through my blood stream I found it hard to get a grip of myself. Usually with my friends around me I'd be at my happiest but that wasn't the case this time. I, for one drunken reason or another, was only wearing my boxer shorts and I wanted to go outside. Part of me found the idea amusing but a large part of me was feeling experimental. I told Michael, who wasn't as drunk as everyone else, that I was going out to get some fresh air. He insisted on joining me, as he could see what a mess I was. We sat on the doorstep of my dad's apartment building talking about my feelings as they had dipped. I wasn't making much sense in the state I was in and my consciousness was very blurry and unstable. The fresh air didn't help that much and I decided to stand up and walk into the road. I could see a car coming and I walked off the pavement and into the road. It was all happening so slowly due to my state but the alcohol made it easy to avoid any hesitation in what I was doing. The car got nearer and before I could put myself in danger Michael ran out and grabbed me only to drag me back to the pavement. The car stopped for a moment then drove onward. I continued to feel miserable after that, I felt like I had ruined my own party. I laid down on a mattress wishing all the bullshit in my life would end, until I fell asleep. I then threw up the following morning and the rest of the day. What a crazy night. At least I found it amusing that I went out into the middle of the road only wearing my underwear.

July, the following month, started off pretty shitty; Charlotte and I had broken up recently. Before we split up I was sticking to my plan of killing myself but she had other ideas. She told me she no longer wanted to die because she was happy with me and wanted to keep going. I was in two minds about this because I loved being with her but hated nearly everything else in my life. When she told me that she no longer wanted to die with me I went along with it. I was infatuated by her and wanted to be with her so I put suicide on hold for the time being. But it didn't matter because she broke up with me some time after that anyway. I didn't take it very well at all. You can only imagine what I did to myself in the evenings to punish myself. I blamed myself for the break up, wishing that I had done better and had been more appealing.

The real kick in the teeth came when my close friend Richard and her got together shortly after. Maybe some of you reading this know how it feels to have a good friend of yours date one of your ex-partners? It can hurt a lot. At the time I put on a brave face in front of them, pretending that it was okay and that I felt nothing. It was hard to hide. I didn't have a problem with them dating it was just painful to see and think about. I never acted malicious but I did make the mistake of having them over one evening to stay at my Mum's house.
We were actually having fun when they came over until we went to sleep. I struggled to sleep generally because destructive and anxious thoughts plagued my mind whilst I would try to fall asleep but having the two of them round made it worse. We slept on mattresses in the front room and whilst I was fighting my emotions they slept in each other's arms peacefully. The sight of the two of them made me feel jealous and broken hearted. I couldn't sleep and I was beating myself up for fucking up my relationship with Charlotte. I knew that the only way to get some sleep was to cut myself and get my endorphin fix. I had used self-harm as a way of getting to sleep when feeling anxious and depressed before so I had to do it again. I went to the kitchen and took a small knife to my wrist. I didn't go over the top as I didn't want any blood to be found, nor did I want them to find out, so, I slept with something on that covered my wrist.

Nearer the middle of the month my suicidal thoughts began to intensify to a level that I had not yet experienced and I decided to give suicide another shot. I was still pretty cut up, excuse the pun, over not being with Charlotte and this was distracting me along with the other pressures and challenges that I was putting up with. I never seemed to be pleasing anyone even though I was spending at least half of my time trying to please everyone. I couldn't figure out what the hell I was supposed to do to please my Mum and Nigel. I was reluctant in leaving the house out of fear of being verbally or physically abused and bullied. The coursework and academic workload was getting on top of me. I enjoyed the subjects but I had no motivation to do any of it. I was distancing myself from my friends, not on purpose, because I knew the end was near for me. Not long after having Richard and Charlotte over Richard called me up one weekend and told me that I had changed, that I was no longer the friend I used to be to him. I had nothing to defend myself with because I knew he was right. I was different, my priorities and desires were different, my mental attitude was different and my behaviours were far from appealing.

I couldn't go on any more. I had enough of dragging people down and feeling like a useless pile of shit every day.

In the middle of July, on a Wednesday, I woke up feeling numb as ever but a little satisfied. Before getting out of bed I laid there for a minute or so and decided today is going to be the day. The day where I would end it, and I mean really end it. No jokes, no attention, no cries for help; just plain old suicide. I got out of bed feeling half decent and half miserable. Miserable because I hated life but decent because I was going to put an end to it today. I got myself ready for Sixth Form as usual. I got the bus and travelled to school as usual. I met my friends and chatted about meaningless things as usual. Everyone was completely clueless as to my intentions. I went to all my lessons and did the same old things. I pretended to be my usual self, which meant trying to be funny at every opportunity and then day dreaming about pain in between my awful jokes. But when I got to the final lesson of the day I decided to try and meet with Charlotte one last time, for the reasons of telling her my feelings once more and to say goodbye. I knew what I was going to do would put her in emotional discomfort but that didn't bother me. Not because I wanted some form of revenge or sick satisfaction but because dying was my priority and I wouldn't let anything stop me.
I sent her a text to meet me after school and come with me to the town where I had made a failed attempt on top of the local shopping centre a few months prior. I prayed that she would accept my invitation. I also didn't want to be alone in the build up to ending my life, because it was scary. Suicide, as appealing as it came across to me at the time, still frightened me. I had a plan but what if things didn't go the way I planned? What if I screwed up? Not to mention the people I'd be leaving behind. Charlotte replied saying she was unsure but I managed to convince her to join me.

During the last lesson of the day, which was an I.T. lesson, I felt a rush of excitement and nervousness run through me. It was hard to hold it together whilst my tutor was attempting to hold my attention. I did my best to try and seem interested and enthusiastic, I even went up to him at the end of the lesson and asked him about the homework that he had assigned us. It was all a part of keeping up an appearance, something that I had plenty of practice at.
Once the day was over I waited on the school field for Charlotte to emerge from her form room. She came out and I gave her a hug like I

usually did to all my friends. We made way towards Chatham, where the shopping centre was waiting for me, and Charlotte seemed suspicious. She had every reason to be. I had not being in regular contact with her since her relationship with Richard and I hadn't met up with her to hang out for a while. Unlike most people who knew me she knew and recognised my depressive and suicidal behaviours. She asked me outright if I was planning on killing myself today so I lied to her because I knew she would back away from me if I did, or worse, call the police. I didn't want to jeopardise my chances.
Eventually we got to this grassy embankment by the back of the shopping centre, which had a bridge that directly lead to the roof. I was beginning to get more and more anxious and I couldn't hold back this weird grin on my face. To anyone who knew what was going on I probably looked crazy, and, I felt pretty crazy. Here I was sitting on a grass patch with my ex-girlfriend, about to commit suicide and I had a big smile on my face. Charlotte knew what was going on by this point. I confessed that I was going to commit suicide right here and that this was goodbye. In a frustrated and concerned tone she asked me why I was doing this. I explained that my feelings about life haven't changed and that as every day passes I feel worse and worse. I told her that every event and experience that causes me to think and feel negative thoughts keep building up inside of me and I can't take it any more. This was the truth. I couldn't do it any more. I also made it clear to her that I still "loved", as much as any teenager thinks they do, her and that I still wanted to be with her. She couldn't be with me and I understood and respected that, although it still hurt.
We had been sitting and talking for at least half an hour and I could feel my stomach going funny. I felt nauseous and shaky. To try and calm my nerves I put on some music on my phone for us to listen to, a song that Charlotte and I had listened to many times because it was depressive and good to headbang to. As soon as it started playing she told me to turn it off. I didn't want to because it reflected my mood and I wanted to hear it one last time.
It wasn't much longer before Charlotte was due to be picked up by her Mum and I was due to run away. Charlotte was receiving texts from her mum telling her to come and get picked up at a car park near bye. She was panicking and begged me not to do it. Every time I refused she kept saying, "please don't". We cuddled and I started to feel some guilt but I had already made up my mind. Adrenaline was taking over my body. Everything seemed to get more intense than it already was.

It was time. I left all my possession with Charlotte and I said goodbye to her. Then I ran. I ran as fast as I could. I ran, ironically, like my life depended on it, towards the roof. As I ran over the bridge I could hear Charlotte shouting, "NO!" I didn't stop or look back at what was behind me, only taking serious action towards ending myself mattered.

In a very short time I had reached the corner of the roof of the shopping centre. The roof was a car park for the shopping centre and there were barely any cars there, maybe two or three in the section that I was in. It was a hot and sunny afternoon, quite in contrast to the mood in which I was in. The cold and miserable rain was a good representation for my regular thoughts and feelings. I sat on the floor up against the short wall that covered the edging to the roof. The wall was short enough for me to climb and jump from as it was only waist high. I guess suicides weren't very common up here. I looked over the edge and down to the ground to see what awaited me at the bottom. It was a different spot to the one that I had previously been to with my friends, this one was a tad higher and there wasn't any traffic below. Below me was a barrier for the car park, a few bushes, a fence and lots of concrete flooring. It looked clear enough for me to hit the concrete directly when the time came, I wouldn't hit anything on the way down. After checking down below I looked around at my other surroundings. To my right on the corner of the roof was a stair well, which I checked constantly out of fear that someone would intercept me. To my left was just a view of the streets and behind me was an empty car park. I felt so paranoid and it caused me to look around over and over again. My anxiety was high and adrenaline was causing me to shake like a leaf. Before I could even look over the edge again I kept thinking that someone would come by and talk to me to stop me. A few cars came in and out of the car park and when they did I slowly walked away from the edge hoping that they wouldn't notice me comprehending jumping to my death. I thought every single car coming my way was an undercover police officer that was going to take me away. But they weren't, when they went away I walked back to the edge again. After sitting there fidgeting for about twenty minutes I got up and started staring over the edge to psyche myself up. It was a long way down to the ground. I felt nauseas and anxious just looking down at the ground. To help try and calm my nerves I jumped about and did some stretches like I used to when I did Ju-Jitsu. I then looked over the edge once more to convince myself that it was the right thing to do and that I wasn't a coward. I looked up and out towards the town and all I could think about was my family and friends, only the good that I saw in them. I felt warm and a little more at peace. “NO! I can’t let myself remember these false representations,” I thought. As much as I knew that my friends and family loved me I kept trying to believe that they’d be better off without me as I stared blankly over the edge at the ground.

After thirty minutes of doing nothing but thinking I was getting frustrated with myself. I wanted to die but it was getting hard to take action. Every time I thought about dying and all the reasons why I wanted to die my brain kept on countering with happy memories and the words, “what if it gets better?” I was so uncomfortable being in my body at that moment. A battle of survival and suicide was raging inside me. For a moment I was going to walk away but I heard another car coming my way so I panicked and climbed over on the short wall and sit with my legs dangling over the edge. After all the shit I had been through I didn’t want to go back. I couldn’t take another day of misery. Not another experience of being bullied or hassled or criticised. I looked back to see if a car was coming but it was just my paranoid mind playing tricks on me. I didn’t move though, I stayed on the edge looking down and thinking. “I could jump any moment,” I joked to myself. “I can do this, I can do this, I *CAN* DO THIS!” I aggressively whispered to myself. My breathing was getting slower and my heart was beating so fast I couldn’t concentrate on what was happening. I kept looking down at the ground, then up again, then down and my thoughts were all over the place. I wanted to cry but I couldn’t for some strange reason. “I need to do this!” I affirmed passively.
Time was ticking and I felt like I had been up there for a short period but I’d actually been there for about forty five minutes. I turned round to see if they were any cameras watching me, the paranoia of being seen was starting to stress me out. I can’t even describe the abundance of negative emotions I was feeling at this time. Back and forth between depressed and anxiety, paranoia and anger, fear and jealousy, stress and frustration. It was like every unpleasant feeling I had up until now was trying to fight each other to gain my attention.
I kept looking down at the ground and visualised myself jumping, then I slowly started thrusting my body forward to try and get some momentum. In my head I was screaming, “I CAN FUCKING DO THIS!” “But my family and friends, could I leave them all? Of course, I could couldn’t I? Yes, no, yes, no.” I was beginning to have second thoughts about killing myself but when I looked back I could see the CCTV cameras moving, I

knew I was being watched. I then thought, "I can't turn back now, they'll put me away." I tried leaning over the edge again but I struggled to get any further than that. I felt afraid, afraid of dying but more afraid of returning to my "regular" life after this incident.
I stood next to the edge and now all I could think about was how my Mum and Step Dad would judge me, this was worse and more serious than last time and that didn't go down well with them so I knew this would send them over the edge, so to speak.

"Fuck sake," I said to myself in frustration. I looked over the edge once more and accepted the fact that I couldn't do it. Feeling disappointed in myself I walked away. With each step I took I could feel the nerves calming and my breaths were try getting back to their usual rate. But the misery was still there. My head was low and the floor was the only thing I could look at. The misery was there because I knew the life ahead of me was going to be different, very different, but I had no idea what that even looked like. But I was about to find out. As I looked up a police car pulled up to me just before I could even get off the roof and behind it was my Mum's car. I stopped to brace myself for whatever was about to come my way and I said nothing. My Mum got out and ran to me to give me the cuddle I needed about an hour ago. With that I got in her car, after she spoke with the police officers, and we drove home. The journey home was less awkward in comparison to the one I had with Nigel the first time I had made an attempt. He was more sympathetic this time and it was nice to get through to him. I always wanted my Step Dad to have more of an understanding of my emotional difficulties and I believed this was a step in the right direction. I wish it could have been achieved less dramatically though. When we got home my mum made us all some pasta, even though I had not eating for about five hours I couldn't eat much. Depression and other low feelings have a tendency to kill off any appetite. I asked to be excused and went to my room to be alone with my thoughts, I couldn't bear to talk to anyone about the afternoon I had just had. Fortunately they were prepared to leave it till the morning.

Chapter 7 – My First Week in a Mental Health Ward

My second attempt at suicide had led to several changes in my life, very significant changes. First of all my Mum finally agreed it was time for me to be on anti-depressants. I don't think she liked the idea of one of her

children having this level of problems but she knew I needed more help than I was getting. We also agreed that my counsellor needed to change as the woman who I had being seeing clearly wasn't working out. The doctor started me on a low dose of gateway anti-depressants, I use the term "gateway" as most people who have my level of emotional difficulties start on them.
Secondly I had stopped Sixth Form, I didn't need any academic pressure hanging over me whilst trying to recover. Honestly, I hated attending education because of how much it consumed me and made me do things I didn't want to do. I still didn't know what I wanted to do with my life and I felt that school wasn't going to help me at this time. I already missed my friends though. I knew I wasn't going to see most of them any more because of where I lived and I wasn't even sure they wanted to see me badly enough, not after what Richard said to me about that fact that I had changed too much. Those words still haunted me.
Word about my attempt at life had got round to pretty much everyone overnight but it didn't bother me. At least most of my friends did care enough to send me messages wishing me well. Things like that made all the difference to me in dark times. Charlotte even returned my belongings that I left with her just before I abandoned her at the shopping centre.

Thirdly, this was the biggest of all changes, I had decided to move in with my Dad. I never thought I'd move in with my Dad due to the childish arguments we had every time I spent time with him. We hadn't been that close since not long after he and my Mum split up some nine years previous. In the last couple of years, since my Dad got made redundant, he had changed, from my perspective at least, which was a good and a bad thing for me. At times he was fun, open minded (he was totally fine with me being bi-sexual) and let me get away with things that I couldn't do at home with my Mum and Nigel such as smoke, drink and talk more openly with a wild sense of humour. But on the other hand he was childish, not very fatherly and liked to drink daily. It was an easy option for me however because I couldn't stand another minute living at home. I felt out of place from that side of my family, like I wasn't meant to be there. I was the typical black sheep. Everyone else was happy, cosy and close where I was miserable, in emotional discomfort and distant. Plus I was getting into an argument or facing criticism virtually every day.

Upon moving in with my Dad I quickly learnt that things weren't quite how I'd expected them to be, but, looking back I think I was just deluded to believe it was going to be an easy ride. He got me to clean his flat daily, nothing to strenuous but enough to make him and I argue over missing a spot of dust or two. I also slept on a mattress that was cut from his old sofa, it was thin and hadn't been washed. It wasn't very comfortable and I woke up most morning with a sore shoulder or back.
I still had my job at the restaurant, not that it helped my emotional health. I got myself into a stupid incident which resulted in me receiving a disciplinary from a high up person in the company. I deserved the disciplinary but I couldn't handle the verbal lashing I received that day. After it was over I walked calmly to the staff toilets and cut at my legs with a steak knife that I grabbed on the way up.

It wasn't all bad though, in contrast it felt easier than living back home. I felt a little freer and closer to my friends. I could finally meet up with them without taking a bus or relying on my folks to drop me off. Though I had a pretty frustrating incident when meeting up with a good friend of mine called Jamie. It was a rainy day in Rochester and we were in the high street, about ten minutes away from my Dad's place. Jamie and I sat under an arch about a quarter of the way down the high street to avoid the rain. We wanted to be out and about, not stuck in doors. Jamie was far less alternative than I was back then and his upbringing was different than mine but we had been good friends for about five years so meeting up was a must, whatever the weather.
The rain was hitting quite hard and it was cold. We remained under this arc for at least half an hour, hoping that the rain would stop anytime soon. I didn't want my hair to get ruined most of all. There was fewer and fewer people around as the rain started to intensify but one girl walked passed us and said, "Hello." Jamie and I responded with the same greeting and the girl smiled and walked off. The girl, who seemed very friendly, was about our age, maybe a year or two younger.
Thirty seconds or so passed before a boy approached us. I was sitting there and only looked at his feet out of fear that he was going to be trouble, and I was right. The boy, lad or whatever you want to call him, dickhead was appropriate too, questioned us and said, "Why did you speak to my sister!?" I was enjoying my day with Jamie until this moment and I started to feel self-loathing again, though, I wasn't feeling anxious like I usually did in moments of confrontation.

I couldn't believe what this boy was asking me and just after he had finished questioning us I looked up to see his face. I couldn't believe it. It was the same guy who threatened and verbally abused me at the end of the previous year when I had tried to enjoy a night out bowling with friends.
Now my anxiety started to take over. I silently prayed that he didn't recognise me otherwise I was fucked. I looked him in the eye and confidently said, "Your sister said hello to us and we said hello back like any polite person would." This logic was not in line with his motives. He was obviously looking to cause fights with weak and "different" looking people like me. He didn't give any indication that he recognised me so I remained calm and I felt more confident than usual, mostly because we were in public and there was more people around than last time. Plus he only had two girls and a guy about his height, and even skinnier than me, with him. Had the need to defend myself arise I felt confident enough to knock him down a notch. Violence was still not a part of me so I did my best to avoid it. This low life told me to get up and fight him, it was like history repeating itself. I said no as usual, he repeated himself, I then responded with the same answer as usual. He tried tapping me with his foot to make me stand up and I refused. I had a feeling he wasn't feeling as confident as he was last time he threatened me. Finally he said aggressively, "Get up or I'll kick you in the face." He couldn't do anything to me that wasn't already worse than what I had been doing to myself so I said, "Go on then." He paused for a second, I could tell he was hesitating. He then turned all of his attention to Jamie and said, "You don't look scared." Jamie was way more confident in these circumstances than I was and responded with a sarcastic, "I'm not." I wanted to laugh so hard at this little shit because he wasn't getting very far with us. Like last time I realised that he was only going to fight if someone made the first move, like the coward that he was.
When words were no good the male friend of this guy walked over to us, whilst the girls stayed back, and tried pushing and shoving Jamie in the chest and demanded that they fight. Other than Jamie being shoved a bit it was hilarious to watch because they obviously set out to fight people who hit them first so they could claim self-defence if they got caught by the police. Typical fucking cowards. I knew that if either of these boys were alone they wouldn't have the balls to pick a fight with anyone.
After a minute of pointless chit chat and shoving I suggested to Jamie that we move on, and the two lads and lasses had the cheek to call us pussies as we walked towards my Dad's flat in the rain.

"Just another day in my shitty life," I thought to myself.

After a couple of weeks I got used to living with a different routine and different rules to the ones I had at my Mum's house. My Dad went out to work his labour job during the day and I had the flat to myself. Now that I didn't go to school and I took a little time off of work I had time to relax and escape all the pressure that I couldn't handle. It was extremely relieving to have no academic pressure and to not have my Mum or Step dad pressure me into trying to figure my life out. I still had no idea what my life was all about and I definitely had no idea what I was going to do long term with myself. I was living moment to moment and hoping that everything would work out, either that or I would make another attempt on my life. But this feeling of relief was short lived and it wasn't long before I found myself getting up to my old habits; cutting.

Monday to Friday, and even on Saturdays, my Dad would get up and go to work before I could even wake up fully. I usually went to bed feeling miserable and questioning if moving in to my Dad's place was a good idea. My Dad and I got on well most of the time but there was a t least one childish argument between us a day, half the time it appeared that he had the same mental age as me, probably because he drank daily. When my Dad left for work in the mornings I'd lay in and try to get back to sleep but once I gained consciousness my imagination and memory faculties would start doing their thing to make me feel depressed. The fact the flat was empty upon me waking up made me feel empty inside. No one to talk with to take my mind off of my painful memories or prevent my imagination from running wild with disturbing creations. Waking up to silence was never a good thing after going to sleep feeling like a sack of shit. When my Dad left I found myself sitting in the bathroom with my razor blades and lashing out on my wrists and legs to relieve the sadness that dwelled within me. I just felt so lonely. I couldn't meet with my friends during the week because they would still be at Sixth Form or school. I sat in silence just thinking too deeply most of the time. When I did cut I tried to be careful to keep my Dad from noticing, which wasn't hard because he was either at work or in the pub that was only two doors down from his front door. They say, "Be careful what you wish for because you might just get it," I had wished for isolation and freedom but now I felt like a prisoner of my own mind. With no one around most of the time I just indulged in my own misery.

In the time between standing on the edge of a shopping centre car park roof and living with my Dad I had to see some mental health professionals who I had offered me support and said that if I was ever going to be a threat to myself then I should call them and they would put me in a "safe place", meaning a mental health ward. At first when they told me this I said that I would be fine, which I wasn't but the idea of going to a hospital ward didn't appeal to me. I imagined the hospital ward to be filled with freaks and crazy people, as much as I was different from the average person I didn't want to be in there. But as each day went by living with my Dad I was still struggling to feel happy or at least content. It was okay at first but the novelty of more freedom had worn off so quickly and I was tearing myself apart so much so that I was considering suicide again.
I told my Dad this one afternoon in his tiny kitchen with the ugly beige walls, I told him that I hated being alive and that I wanted to die still, I told him with anger and frustration in my voice because half the time it felt like I couldn't get through to him. But he did take this in. For the first time ever he was speechless, usually he had something to say about everything but this time he had nothing to say. He looked at me and his eyes started to well up. I hadn't seen my Dad cry since our holiday in Brazil seven years earlier. He couldn't string his words together properly but I could tell he wanted to help me. I had always loved my Dad, despite his poor efforts at parenting and the fact he was the cause of him and my Mum breaking up nine years ago, and this was the first time in years that I had seen his emotional side. I told him about going into hospital for some extra support and help with my recovery then he helped make the phone call. Once again I asked myself, "Am I doing the right thing?" A lot of the time I struggled to determine what the right thing to do was.

I spent the next few hours gathering my things and mentally preparing myself. All I had been told was that a "bed" was waiting for me. It was an ominous thought. What kind of bed? Would this bed be amongst other beds in a ward? What kind of people would I be mixing with? I hated going into the unknown because my anxiety would cause a million questions to start running through my head, questions that I couldn't answer truthfully and my imagination always seemed to come up with the worst possible outcomes for me. I wasn't proud to being going in to hospital for mental health issues. I already felt weird for seeing a therapist on and off and taking anti-depressants. But going into hospital was a big step up on the nutcase spectrum. Strangely enough, when the time came to leave for hospital I felt less anxious than I had done when I was told I was being admitted. I felt satisfied with my decision because it was another way of escaping reality, something that I was always trying to do. I hoped that going into hospital was going to feel like a holiday for my mind and emotions, that way I may have a better chance at coping with myself and my life.

We arrived at the hospital in the afternoon, about half past one I think it was. My Dad came with me to the mental health area of the hospital and we were seen by some of the staff there. A middle age woman with blonde hair had told us to wait whilst the arrangements for my stay were being finished. My Dad and I waited in the waiting room. I had already been to this waiting room a few times before when waiting to be assessed by specialists after I made suicidal threats. It was a wide and bright room, out of the windows you could see an internal hospital garden of some sort but the one thing that made this room uncomfortable was this strange noise. It was off-putting for someone like me. The noise went on for a long time, repeating every few seconds. The only way I can describe this noise was that it sounded like someone who was shrieking in emotional turmoil. Every ten seconds you could hear, "Agghhh," over and over and over again. In my mind I saw someone in the mental health ward clawing at a window making this noise with a face of agony. But I told myself that it was the air conditioning or something so that I could remain calm. I had dreams about mental wards before and none of them were pleasant, I just wanted my stay to be as comfortable as possible.

The blonde haired woman returned eventually and told my Dad and I to follow her up to the ward. Now I was starting to panic. We followed the woman who walked very slowly for some reason, which didn't help. I wanted to quickly get in and get settled. What seemed like a long and slow walk was only a few minutes long and we arrived at the front door to the ward. Like all the wards in the hospital this door required a special key card to get in, or you buzzed the intercom to get someone to let you in. My heart was racing as we went through the front door. In my mind I hoped that there would be some troubled teens, or at least one, that I could talk to and connect with. That hope was quickly shot down, as we walked to the main reception desk I looked around at this L shaped ward and noticed that everyone was at least ten years older than me. Some of the patients were as old as pensioners and were obviously not mentally fit to be out in society. I could see an older women talking with herself whilst the others congregated in what resembled a living room.

The staff that were walking around seemed very calm and friendly so I thought that this may work out. Once I had signed some paperwork a member of staff then showed me to my room. Unlike the other patients I had my own room due to my age. I was still afraid of what might happen here so at least I had some privacy if I needed it. I walked into the room and it had navy walls with a small window that didn't open very far, for obvious reasons. As I turned back round to face the door I noticed that a previous occupant had scribed a rather large message into the plaster wall above the bed that covered most of the wall. It said some along the lines of, "Mummy and Daddy don't love me." I had this haunting flash of someone like me being forced into this room and taking their anger out on the wall. I was curious as to how they had written this message on the wall as the staff banned anything that was sharp. The staff had to look after those kinds of possessions.
After dumping my belongings in the room I was shown to the canteen and was told the times we ate. My Dad seemed welcoming of the experience and tried his best to verbally comfort me. Perhaps he felt guilty that he couldn't look after me well enough?
Now that the guided tour had finished it was time to say goodbye to my Dad. We went to my new room and he told me that he would visit and contact me daily. Even though I wanted to escape my regular life I was glad that he showed some compassion; not something he showed me much of.
Once my Dad left, which wasn't a very nice feeling, I sat in my room and messaged Charlotte to tell her where I was. I don't know why I was messaging her, I probably wanted her attention and sympathy. I never usually wanted people's attention and sympathy because people who self-harmed received an unnecessary bad reputation for being attention seeking, so I did my best to be the opposite. But I still had some feelings for Charlotte so I went ahead and messaged her.

Other than texting Charlotte, which was limited due to my lack of phone credit, I just sat there staring at the walls and ceiling of my dingy room. I felt like I was alone in my Dad's flat again but this time I had people watching me. After a couple of hours of staring blankly into nothing there was a knock at my door. One of the mental health nurses asked me what I wanted for dinner. The options sounded surprisingly tasty. I hadn't eating anything in hours and my Dad didn't make much effort in cooking so I guess any meal sounded good. Another hour or so passed and another knock came at the door, this time dinner was being served. I walked down the corridor and on the right, opposite the reception desk was the canteen. There was about six or so tables spread out on the right whilst the serving hatch was to the left. Like a typical new kid in school I sat by myself as I had no interest in making friends with the other patients. I convinced myself that I wasn't as "crazy" as they were, not that I was judging. I ate my meal quickly and moved on to dessert. Once that was devoured I was still hungry, fortunately the server behind the hot counter offered me a second sponge pudding.

Dinner was as exciting as my first day got. I spent most of it in my room holding onto my duvet waiting for time to pass and thinking of what would happen once I got out, and then questioning how long I'd actually be in here as no one told me how long that would be. Days? Weeks? Months? It was horrible not knowing how long I'd be in this depressing place. At least I was safe from the things that emotionally and physically harmed me on the outside world.
At around ten that evening another knock came, this time it was time for medication. We were made to get in line at the medicine hatch. I had images of those films and TV shows where mental patients line up and get forced to take pills when they refused. Everyone in my line was well behaved. After taking my pill I went back to my room to try and get some sleep. Doing nothing all day but thinking and staring blankly was exhausting believe it or not. That's the thing with depression, you don't have the energy you normally have. Even doing nothing makes you more tired than usual. I got into my pyjamas, usually I only wore my underwear but doing that felt a little awkward here. My Mum and Dad then called me one after the other to ask how I was and how my stay was going, I had nothing to say other that the usual; "It's fine." I said that about everything that made me fell low to avoid further conversation about it. I missed them, as well as all my friends, and I started to feel depressed very intensely. It was so lonely here. I tried to lay down and closed my eyes but I couldn't stop thinking about my situation. I pictured myself in this unusual place and comparing myself to the other people that were in here. I then thought about Charlotte. Then I thought about a variety of messed up experiences that I had over the past year. I didn't sleep for the first few hours. My mind was racing and I stared at the clock and the walls some more. I didn't fall asleep till about 1am that night.

I got woken around eight by a staff member telling me to get up for breakfast. Being a teenager eight o'clock was far too early for me, and, being depressed meant that it was even harder to drag myself out from under the comfy duvet of this hospital bed. After five minutes of trying to motivate myself I made way to the canteen for breakfast. I rarely ate anything after waking up but I knew that meals were hours between each other so I had to make the most of the cereal that was available. Again, I sat alone trying not to make eye contact with the other patients. But they seemed to get along, they spoke to one another like they were best friends. "Maybe I should start to make friends?" I thought. Once breakfast was out of the way I was expected to sit around and be bored for the foreseeable future. The ward was extremely boring, and, ironically, it was enough to drive you crazy. I hadn't even been in this place for twenty four hours and it was beginning to get to me. It's like the environment I was in was magically massaging my brain with disturbing thoughts and trying to get me to crack. As I sat in my room waiting for something to happen I convinced myself that I wasn't like these other people. For the next few hours I sat on my bed listening to depressing music. I had made a playlist some months back that I listened to when I felt depressed or when I was cutting myself. I know that sounds messed up but at the time it felt like something I needed.

At midday I went to lunch and continued to sit alone, but this time I looked around at everyone to try and learn something about them. I wanted to know their names and understand what mental or emotional problems they had so I could work out if I could potentially make a temporary friendship with them. All of them were older than me but I wanted someone to talk to. This place was lonely, as much as it was full of people I felt more alone than ever.

In the afternoon I had to have a blood test, the first one I've had in years. I wasn't afraid of needles, after all, cutting yourself with a razor blade is more painful, right? The blood test was a lot more draining, literally, than I remembered from previous ones. They took three syringes worth of blood and by the third one I was feeling light headed, so much so that I had to be practically carried back to my room. Upon getting back to my room I threw up in my bin where I felt so dizzy. One of the staff gave me some orange juice to perk me up but I was ready to pass out for some time. It was easier to be asleep during my tedious stay here.

I woke up about two hours later to find that it was visiting time. Unlike most of the other wards visiting hours were very short in my ward. Perhaps they didn't want the patients to get too attached to their loved ones and start going "crazy", excuse the terrible pun. My Mum and Dad came to visit me together. It was nice to see them at the same time and it was even better to see them on good terms. Usually when I thought of them together I just had memories of arguments and unpleasant remarks so this was a treat. It was hard to speak to them openly about my feelings with them still. I found myself telling them that I was fine at almost every opportunity, just like I usually did. They asked me questions about the place I was in but I didn't want to talk about it. I never wanted to speak about anything that was related to mental health with my family, it just didn't feel right and I wanted to protect them from the darkness that clouded my mind. Telling my own flesh and blood that I wanted to kill myself wasn't exactly the easiest thing to say, let alone have a full conversation about it. I saved those kinds of words for the professionals. After they went I went back to my room until dinner time. Nothing worth mentioning happened between then and the next morning so let's skip to day three.

The next morning I woke up a little earlier than usual. I sat up and turned round then put my feet on the cold hard floor to find that my slippers had been moved. I looked under my bed and found one of them. I questioned myself whether I had left them together or not. I searched my room for fifteen minutes and was starting to get anxious. Had someone been in my room whilst I was asleep and taken a slipper? This was a mental health ward so anything was possible. I had previously seen some of the other patients talking to themselves for hours so I had to expect the unexpected. I checked my bag that had higher valued items in it to make sure my iPod, wallet and phone were still there, which they were. I couldn't help think how strange it was that someone had taken one slipper and nothing else. I left my room to inform a member of staff that my slipper had gone, they probably thought I was mad for suggesting this. I walked back to my room past one of the older female patients and I could hear my slipper. By "hear my slipper" I mean that it had a button that you pushed and it made a noise. I wasn't sure if I had heard correct so I turned round and followed this woman to make sure. I heard the noise again. Rather than try and reason with this woman, who barely spoke a word in the last couple of days, I asked a member of staff to try and retrieve it. It's not often you ask someone to retrieve your slipper from an older woman's dressing gown. I was confident that the staff had dealt with more peculiar incidents.

After breakfast I was told that we were going to occupational therapy. I had no idea was this meant but everyone else seemed pretty happy about

it. Everyone gathered together, including the patients from the adjoining mental health ward. We all got together and stood as a group whilst they marked us down on a register. I carefully looked round at the patients from the other ward. They seemed louder than the patients in my ward. I instantly came to the assumption that their ward was for people with problems of a more serious nature.
As the register was being done something was said between a little old man, roughly in his seventies or eighties, and a lady in her fifties to sixties that caused a problem. I didn't quite hear what was said but as I looked round this woman smacked the little old man on the top of the head with an open palm. A downward slap if you will. She hit him with some force too. I was shocked at such behaviour, mostly because this old man was so small, skinny and frail. Another patient from the other ward, Ronald, started chuckling and said something to this little old man, who I then found out was called Michael. Ronald chuckled and said something to Michael that I couldn't make out. It was a very fast mumble with a hint of laughter in his voice. The staff quickly defused the situation and we made our way to occupational therapy, whatever that meant.

We reached occupational therapy and it was not what I expected at all. It was like I had entered a room full of "normality" and positivity, quite in contrast to the depressing ward that I had come from. I looked round at this large room like a child in a sweet shop. I could see tables for table tennis, comfy sofas, lots of books & puzzles and a pool table. Outside was a nice size patio with benches, swing ball and an area to play badminton. I was happy to be somewhere that resembled the outside world but it put my situation in perspective and I started to feel down again. I missed the freedom I had before, I use the term freedom loosely as I didn't feel completely free but I was more free than being stuck in a mental health ward. The other patients quickly walked over to their chosen activities and areas of recreation whilst I stood and looked around. I didn't feel comfortable mingling in with the other patients so I drifted around the room slowly waiting for time to pass. After scanning the room from corner to corner I sat down on a chair so I could feel sorry for myself. I was used to this passive action. Feeling sorry for myself was something I tried to avoid so that I didn't match the usual stereotype people judge me for but today I gave in and let myself feel bad. I looked at everyone else having fun and I sat there wishing I was at home. As usual I had my iPod playing sad songs in my ears.

In the afternoon I had a meeting with some of the therapists which meant I was due to tell my life story all over again. It was emotionally draining telling people that you were depressed, self-harming and wanting to kill yourself. The thing is that when you suffer from depression you feel low and lethargic most of the time anyway but when you express your feelings and share your experiences right down to the darkest and most miserable detail you end up feeling like your life has been sucked out of you and you're just left with your body; no heart or soul. That's how I felt every time I walked away from every assessment I ever had with a mental health professional.
The meeting was like every other meeting; I spoke and the therapist did their best to appear empathic, that was my assumption of them anyway. It was hard to tell if they cared or not because I had low expectation of all people. Depression does that unfortunately. I did ask if I was allowed to leave the hospital at any point during my stay, just for a couple of hours. There was a new album by one of my favourite punk bands due to be released the next day and I was desperate to get hold of it. I knew that would help me stay a little calmer during my stay on the ward. To my surprise I was granted a couple of hours leave the next day as long as I was escorted by my Mum. I left that meeting feeling a little happier than usual thanks to the upcoming freedom I was going to get.

Over the next four days very little happened. I have nothing worth sharing with you about the rest of my stay in the mental health ward because every day was practically a repeat of the previous day. You wake up, get breakfast, then get ready for the day, sit round in your room for an hour wishing you were either dead or in a better place, then you went for occupational therapy, then came back for an hour to feel bored or depressed again, then lunch, then a couple of hours before visiting time, then dinner, then another few hours of misery until medication time came and then bed time. It may sound dull, boring and depressing because it is. It's also very tiring. You may think that doing nothing is easy but staying in a place like that is exhausting for your mind. I was lucky to have my own room, most of the other patients shared open beds with nothing more than a curtain separating their private space. When I was told I could leave I almost jumped for joy. Before I went in I expected a break, some isolation from the dangers and fears I had of the rest of the world and people to look after me and that's exactly what I got but I didn't expect it to feel so lonely and depressing. If anyone reading this has

been sectioned or an inpatient then you will know where I'm coming from. "I'm never going back there" I said to myself.
But coming out back into the world wasn't that easy either. I had only been gone for seven days and in that time I spoke to some of my friends friends, a few of them visited me, but now I felt like I had alienated myself from most of my social group and my non-immediate family. If I'm honest with myself I was more afraid of them judging me than anything else. Who wanted to associate with a crazy person like me?

Chapter 8 – A Relationship with Suicide

A week in the mental health ward was a bit of an eye opener for me, I thought that I had better change a few things if was to make the next few months a little more bearable. My first priority was being more clever about hiding cuts on my body, and, hiding my feelings about my life from my friends and family better than I had done previously; no more questions from my loved ones. I wasn't going to tell anyone about the fact I was fantasising about suicide again in case I ended up in the loony bin. My second priority was to get back into my restaurant job to earn some money. I was poor and my Dad barely made enough money to pay for his flat and drinking and smoking habits, more importantly I wanted to do some retail therapy plus I missed going to gigs. I told the restaurant manager, Jo, whom I got on well with, that I was doing better and was ready to return, even though I wasn't that much better, I was just better at hiding the truth. And my third priority was to get back out there and be with friends again, and, maybe find someone to have some sexual fun with. Being isolated in a mental ward was one of the loneliest experiences of my life and I wanted to avoid being lonely again. Don't get me wrong, I needed to be alone from time to time but during the day I needed interaction with people who understood me, or at least I felt comfortable to be myself around. The only time I wanted to be alone was when I was self-harming or feeling super low. Self-harming, as much as my friends and family knew, I had no desire to let them see me cutting. I already felt guilty for self-harming and even guiltier when my loved ones saw the cuts on my wrists, I could only imaging how bad I'd feel if they actually saw me in the act of self-harm.

Weekends were the only times I could see my friends as they were still at school or sixth form and I no longer attended formal education, with the exception of a digital photography class I took once a week at the local library. My Mum and Nigel were far more ambitious and suggestive than my Dad so they continued to push and stretch me to make something for myself, so I made an attempt to try and go down the photography route as it was a subject that I was interested in. Even though I fantasised about suicide there were still parts of me that hoped for a better life. My recent experiences with being on top of a roof contemplating suicide and be trapped in a mental health ward had swayed me to want to live a little more than I did a few months ago. When you go down emotionally you want something to balance you out and the hope of future achievement has the potential to give you a little more strength to keep going on. I only realised this many years later.

I made a lot of effort to see my friends where possible, and I had plenty of friends to see. I made a lot of friends whilst in secondary school and even more friends whilst at Sixth form, mostly with girls of the lower year groups. I found it challenging to make friends with people of my exact age or older due to my confidence, with people a year or two younger than me I felt more comfortable.

I found myself trying to hang out with Charlotte to get on reasonable friendship terms again, she still meant something to me and I wanted to at least be in her company. I also had another female friend named Leanne, whom I had gone to a concert with in February earlier that year. I spent a lot of time with Jamie and Michael too. Through all these friends I had I made friends with their group of friends and we all hung around in Rochester, as that was the place to be, rain or shine.

We had a very unfortunate event one afternoon in Rochester that still sticks with me and nearly gets me boiled up every time I think about it, but for you the reader I will share this story.

Charlotte, Leanne, Michael, two other friends of mine, Laurence and Jake, and I were hanging around as usual in Rochester in an area known as "The Vines". It was like a small park that had plenty of grass, light grey gravel paths and very old black iron & wood benches. The park was long and narrow and was away from the town centre and any main roads, with lots of trees on the outer edges. If you saw it you would imagine yourself going for a jog or walking your dog down there. We usually hung around the Rochester castle grounds but it was busy there and we wanted to be away from all that. It was about 4pm and we had been having a lovely day but our positive emotions were about to be compromised. An old friend of mine from primary school, who was also a friend of Leanne's, came over to us to warn us about a large group of boys from a notorious and rough road in the next town were down in Rochester looking for "grungers" to beat up. I found the idea amusing, thinking that it was just a handful of young boys until my old friend confirmed there was about twenty to thirty of them. My old friend left us to go home and avoid any problems and the rest of us agreed we should probably do the same. But we sat there for another fifteen minutes or so and in that time I noticed at the other side of the park a guy dressed in a tracksuit standing alone staring in our direction. I could feel panic manifesting in my stomach, I had a strong feeling this guy was a part of the large group of thugs that my friend had spoken of. And I was right.

I made the rest of our group aware of what I saw and we quickly agreed it was time to get our asses out of there. I suggested we moved swiftly but didn't act as scared as we actually was. But before we knew it the one lad that I saw in the distance alerted his friends, if you can honestly call them that, by shouting, "there they are, get them!" That was it. At that point my stomach dropped and both anxiety and adrenaline started to rush like lightning through my body. From round the corner, where the "spotter" was standing, came at least twenty other boys. We started to run in the opposite direction in complete panic. I could feel the fear in my friends, as well as my own fear. I knew I could run fast, having run a lot in PE at school, but I was under the impression my friends were fairly slow compared to me. Michael, Jake and Laurence at the time were larger builds than me, I was still a skinny 30 inch waist, which meant I could outrun them quite easily and I did run past them very quickly. I knew if anyone was going to get caught it would be them. I didn't feel proud of running away quicker than them but under the circumstances I had very little choice.
We got out of the park within seconds and I suggested we split up, and, in a panicking tone I demanded that Charlotte and Leanne knock on a door of a house to get help.
We were in an area that was near the high street but in an irrational move I ended up running towards houses and pubs. But these weren't the kind of houses that had people coming in and out of all the time, nor were the pubs open at this hour, it just seemed like there were no adults in sight at all and the more I ran through this adult-less street the more I began to feel sick with anxiety and panic. I didn't look back to see where my friends were but I could hear the sound of Michael, Laurence and Jake running and shouting towards me. I couldn't make out what they were saying, all I

could focus on was making it to a hiding spot and waiting for time to pass. I honestly believed I could outrun them but fear was getting the better of me.
After running for what seemed like only a few minutes I ran past a driveway that had an arc over the entrance so I took my chances and stopped to go through. I didn't care if this place was private property, I just wanted to make it to the end of the day without being beaten the shit out of.
I looked round and there wasn't anywhere to climb or any doors to anyone's house. But there was a ditch at the end of the driveway. The ditch was actually an old alley way of some sort that had been blocked at both ends. This ditch, was about ten meters long, about two meters wide and just under two meters deep. I jumped in the ditch to hide, it was only a minute or so before Jake and Laurence jumped in behind me. I pulled myself up the wall on the other side of the ditch to see if we could climb it and escape that way but to my disappointment instead was a very steep slope, practically vertical, that lead onto the backs of houses. The drop was too high to make safely but it didn't stop me contemplating it. I wondered what would be worse; having my face smashed in or potentially damaging my legs and ankles from a twenty foot drop. I decided to stay put and pray that they wouldn't find us.

Laurence, Jake and I were panting loudly trying to catch our breath but at the same time trying to suppress it so we wouldn't be found. I whispered to them asking where Michael went but they weren't sure. The floor beneath us was muddy and we were surrounded by stinging nettles in this old alleyway ditch thing. In the few minutes that we waited I was trying to work out how far the gang of boys would be in relation to us, I didn't want to poke my head up and see if they had walked past or not, for all I knew they were nearby and I didn't fancy risking it for my friends and me.
I had a feeling that they had not past us yet so we kneeled down in the dirt and tried to stay quiet. After being in silence in this ditch for about five minutes I heard running coming towards us and before I could put two and two together I looked up to see Michael throw himself into the ditch to join us. It was at that moment my stomach dropped even further. Michael was in a more intense state of panic than the rest of us which lead me to believe he had been spotted coming to where we were hiding. I asked him if he had been followed, and I had a strong feeling he had, and in his breathless state he said, "I'm not sure, but I think they saw me." In my head I was frustrated and I couldn't help but think, "Why did you

come this way and lead them to us?" I couldn't ask him that though. Instead I went to pull myself back up to see if the gang had found their way on to this secluded drive way. But before I could stick my head up and look over a boy, no older than ten, stood above us looking down with a big grin, a grin that gave me the impression that things were about to get fucked up, and all he could say was, "hello." I wanted to plea and beg to the boy that he didn't summon his group of friends but I didn't want to come across as a coward. Plus I was shocked that a boy of such a young age was hanging around with such rough low lives. A minute or so passed and before I could think of anything smart to do or say and the ground above our ditch became crowed with the gang of boys.

They stared down on us like vultures waiting for their next meal. With the way I was feeling I could have been bottom of the food chain. I could feel my palms and forehead starting to sweat, not from the summer heat but from the fear and anxiety. My chest pounded harder than it did when I was running away from them and I could feel my arms and hands shaking. I did my best to hold it in as much as possible, I knew from previous experience that bullies went for the most visibly scared victim and I wasn't prepared to be that person today.
They continued to stare down at us four and not a word was said for the first minute. I was standing with my hands in my pockets to the left of us, Laurence to my right, Michael to his right and Jake at the other end. I looked up and noticed the gang were all younger than me and I thought, "great, now I'm about to be beaten up by kids." Their ages varied between roughly between ten and sixteen at the most, what pissed me off the most was the fact I knew I could have had any of them individually but instead they were the real cowards going after people in smaller groups like us.
After a minute, a long minute, had passed some of the boys parted to make way for whom I could only assume was the leader of their group. The oldest, and clearly the only one with balls to make the first move, of their group jumped down into our trap of a ditch and started mocking us for our "grunger" clothes. Oh the verbal abuse was hilarious as always, a narrow minded low life mocking us for wearing clothes that weren't tracksuits or colourful casuals. It was pretty stupid bearing in mind we didn't dress anything like a 90s grunger, no baggy pants, messy long hair or anything resembling Kurt Cobain. The term "grunger" was generally used by ignorant bullies to describe and mock anyone who dressed in alternative clothes. The ring leader, if you like, of the gang said that I

dressed like a faggot, to which I said nothing of course, silence was my best option at this point. He walked up and down us staring at us whilst trying to look as hard as possible. Making us afraid clearly got him going. Some of the other boys above us kept trying to spit on Laurence and successfully got him in the face. The rest joined in on the "grungers are gay and dirty" band wagon. I felt sorry for Jake the most, he was a few years younger than the rest of us and he had only come down to Rochester to visit Laurence, now he was facing a gang of brainless thugs. He pleaded, "Why are you picking on us, we've done nothing wrong?" The response was poor; "We hate grungers," one of the boys replied. With each passing moment I felt myself becoming more anxious and tighter in the chest. My fists were clenched so hard my nails were pinching my palms.

There was no reasoning with these kids and out of nowhere the leader pushed Michael and punched him in the mouth, I could see some blood dripping from his bottom lip as he tried to block his face from further attacks. He then turned to Jake and punched him in the face. Jake started to cry and plea some more whilst the rest of the boys laughed and spat down on us. Laurence was next in line to take a hit to the face, he bled a little and I could see tears in his eyes. It didn't surprise me at all, I probably would have cried if I cared more about my life but the suicidal attitude I had helped me stay partially careless about the who thing, I cared more about my friends than I did myself.
I was next in line for a punch and once the leader was done with Laurence my whole perception went into slow motion. It was the adrenaline I guess and my body knew what was coming. He looked me in the eye for a second before I turned my head to the left and raised my left hand to cover my ear just in time to interception his fist. I had learned and practised that move many times in Ju-jitsu and it came in handy. Unlike my friends I got away lightly with nothing more than a numb ear.

After his attempt to hurt me he walked back towards Michael and demanded that he repeated the words, "I love" followed by a name I will not mention in this book for protection purposes. Michael, in his fearful state, asked him why he should repeat such words and that he will be called "gay" if he does. The leader of the gang quickly edged forward and got up in Michael's face and shouted the same demands again. Michael had no choice but to say, "I love..." etc. etc. It was demoralising to say the least; being told to say that you love a man whom you have no idea who

he is. Although it was fairly obvious that the name this guy was throwing about was his own name, why would you make someone say that they love someone else? This bully was clearly not a smart as he thought he was being, we could now use a name in a police statement at least.
Jake pleaded some more and asked why the gang were doing this to us. As much as I wanted to know why they were being dickheads and trying to scare us I knew all too well that bullies have a motive to feel tough and better than their victims so no amount of questioning, pleading or begging was going to stop them, or even get them to verbally admit their own motives. I knew the boys wanted to feel dominant, and they probably did feel dominant for what felt like a lifetime but was more or less only thirty minutes. But inside I keep thinking, "these boys are idiots if they think this is going to get them anywhere in life." I kept my mouth shut the whole time though.
As Jake continued to ask the same question over and over again, "why are you doing this, we've done nothing wrong?" some of the lads above us spoke of hating grungers, but also admitted that some grungers were alright, which made me laugh a little inside as these boys were too stupid to get to know someone before judging them.
The leading bully continued to walk up and down us some more and pushed us all individually to try and get one of us to fight back, which one of us might have done if he'd been alone, but bullies are too scared to operate alone; they have no back up for one thing and secondly they have no one to impress. This guy was so desperate for one of us to fight back but he was too stupid to realise that we were smart enough to not make a move. He did try and hit Michael again though, this time he managed to block a punch directly to the face. The experience of being trapped was making me feel claustrophobic, something that I never felt before, and I was trying so hard not to burst with anger and into tears. At this moment I accepted this was the worse situation I had ever been in, this is what animals must feel like when their hunted for food and I hated every second of it, though I did have a moment where I fantasised being alone with the gang leader and fighting him. He wasn't much bigger than me, more fat on him than me for sure but no brains to back up his muscle. I couldn't fantasise for long though as I had to dodge spit that was being projected down towards me from time to time. The tension was increasing constantly and whilst the attention was off of me for a moment I wondered when this was going to end, and, how it was going to end. As another boy from the group jumped down to join us I had a flashing image come into my consciousness of the whole group jumping in and

pummelling us until we were unconscious. My hearted raced even faster and sweat was pouring from my forehead. “We’re going to die,” I thought.

Out of nowhere, and just in the nick of time, a voice from the distance shouted “Oi!” The whole group of boys turned around and started slowly walking away. I dared move, neither did my friends, I was too scared to do anything but try and catch my breath and let my tears out a little. I hated crying whilst wearing eye-liner, as I like maintaining my dark and feminine image, but on this occasion I couldn’t care less. A middle age man in a lightly coloured shirt leaned over and asked if we were ok and said it was ok to come out. I almost didn’t believe it though, after that traumatic event anything unpleasant was possible, but I heard Leanne and Charlotte’s voice calling us in the near distance. We climbed out of the pit of doom one by one and I had no idea what my friends were thinking but as I climbed out it felt as if someone had let go of my throat after trying to choke me to death. I didn’t turn around to look back, I just got the fuck out of their and slowly walked towards Leanne and Charlotte for the hug of a lifetime. I put my arms around them and it was fucking emotional. I was yet to hear of what happened to them after we had split off from each other and I didn’t feel like asking, I just wanted to enjoy the friendly cuddle.
Once our cuddle was over I turned around to give some similar affection to Michael, Laurence and Jake, who were expressing a variety of emotions. Michael had tears in his eyes but came across more furious than sad, I could almost feel the clenching of his fists and the grinding of his teeth. He then chuckled a little and said that the guy who appeared to lead the gang, and the one who force Michael to make a false homosexual confession, was a fucking moron for using a full name as it was clearly his own name and that he was going to use the name in a police statement he was going to make once he got home. Michael had always been a clever and caring guy so it was nice to see him expressing some sort of fighting spirit, even though nothing might come from contacting the police.
Once she had wiped her tears away Leanne went on to tell us that her and Charlotte had tried knocking on several doors before anyone answered them and that when they were trying some of the gang boys passed them and frightened them by saying that they were going to rape them. At this point my fists were clenched so tight I could have broken my knuckles. Every time I thought about the bullies and how they tried to get the

better of me I found myself getting extremely wound up to the point where I generally want to hurt someone, as well as myself. Even now, writing about this experience I find myself getting tense from the images in my head.
We walked away together feeling each other's pain and fear, but I felt like somehow it was my fault because I was the one who suggested we all hung out today. I found it easy to blame myself for a lot of things, even when there was no logical reason to. Of course I wasn't to know that we were going to be hunted like prey but I couldn't help believe I was at least partially to blame.

That night I was able to relieve myself of the guilt, as well as the anxiety, and the sadness that came from the day's experience. It wasn't a pretty sight, looking at my left wrist or either of my thighs. Generally speaking the more something affected me emotionally the more I took it out on myself so that I could balance the emotionally tension with physical pain, otherwise I wouldn't be satisfied enough. Whilst living at my Dad's I self-harmed in the living area, which was also my sleeping space, but I could only do so once he went to sleep in his bedroom which was in the next room. I wrapped my duvet around me so if he was to walk in I could hide it quickly. Before we both went to bed I did tell my Dad what happened to me that day and he got more furious than I did but like me he couldn't do anything about it, he had to accept it just like I did.
The next morning I was in pain from the cutting. This happened all the time but this morning was worse, I think it was due to the fact that I felt way shittier, emotionally, than usual. I woke up to the images still being fresh in my mind, which brought an instant feeling of sickness to my stomach and panic to my chest. It was probably a minor for of post-traumatic stress disorder, though I've never been an expert on the subject. My legs weren't too bad, as I had good leg muscles, but my wrist stung like a bitch. When I self-harmed at night I usually slept sleeveless so let air get to the cuts and when I awoke I'd put a long sleeve hoodie or some arm warmers to keep my fresh cuts hidden. That always hurt because fibres from the clothing material would get caught on the scabs, which obviously tugged on the wounds and sent unpleasant messages through my nervous system. I usually felt regret too after self-harming, which was odd because I convinced myself regularly that there was no shame in self-harming.
My Dad had gone to work so I was on my own again. Today was a little more depressing than usual because I struggled to let go of what

happened the day before. I slowly moved around the flat, drifting, and whilst doing so the scenes of the previous day were playing in my mind over and over and over again, like a depressing movie stuck on an infinite loop. Instead of being angry like I was yesterday I felt extremely deflated and low, I couldn't even think straight and make up my mind as to what I should being doing with myself. Different moments of the day came to me one by one; Charlotte and Leanne upset, Michael getting his face smacked, Laurence being spat in the face, Jake pleading for mercy, but, I mostly had the evil look of the gang's faces staring at us, waiting to pounce and make our lives even more miserable. I kept trying to tell myself that I could have avoided this situation, not that that helped at all because I had no way of changing the past.

I didn't even want to go outside, not after that shitty experience. I had been through enough events, some of which I have mentioned in this book, of bullying for me to draw the conclusion that the world was a nasty place and that I was safer to stay in doors for the foreseeable future. The chances were slim but I didn't want to cross paths with any of the people who had verbally or physically abused me before so I stayed in all day, wasting a whole day. That's one of the annoying things about suffering with anxiety; if you experience something awful you assume it's going to happen again even though the chances are slim and it keeps you from doing the things you should be doing. The comfort zone gets smaller and smaller with every undesirable experience.

A week had passed since being chased, threatened and attacked by a gang of boys and I had only left the flat to go to work and to the pub next door with my Dad, even they were struggles but at least they were distractions from the depressive and anxious thoughts that I had that constantly plagued my mind. To get to work I had to walk as fast as I could and walk with my head held high whilst not making eye contact with anyone. The aim was to give off the impression I was confident because I believed that people were more likely to leave me alone. I had the odd comment about my hair or skinny jeans but I was used to it. I didn't wear eyeliner to work in case any narrow minded bullies called me nasty names or threatened to physically harm me, it was easier that way. Going to work was actually good for my well-being, mostly, so I found it easy to motivate myself to go and do it, it was just walking to work that I was afraid of. After what had happened recently who could blame me? Walking to and from work gave me the confidence to hang out with friends and be outside again and this felt like a big achievement for me. It wasn't easy though, I walked around whilst looking over my shoulder and I tried to read people to see if they looked like a potential threat. I stayed away from any groups of "Chavy" looking boys too. I wanted to avoid all confrontation, like I had been doing all my life, and to stay safe. Sometimes I would reflect on this and think, "Why the fuck have I got to be careful when I walk around in public just because I dress differently from the typical tracksuit wearing teenager?" I was never ashamed of being myself but it came at a price. At least I was willing to pay the price even if it meant getting hated for it. I never wanted to change who I was otherwise "they" would win wouldn't they? I was able to meet up with friends on a regular basis again, and, I had made new friends again. The good thing about the alternative community in my area was that everyone wanted to hang around Rochester, especially the castle grounds, in large groups and someone from one group always knew someone else so you ended up meeting so many people. I was quite well known by this point so people usually embraced me with open arms. One of the people in my group was a gay guy called Adam whom I found extremely amusing, his sense of humour was enough to make me go into hysterics. I wasn't looking for a relationship with him, and I had only had one short relationship with a guy previously, but his personality was enough to win me over for some sexual fun.

As it was the summer holidays all of my friends were on a break from school or Sixth form so I could see them almost every day, which helped me gain full confidence in leaving my Dad's flat and being outside for hours on end without feeling anxious or fearful. I had been hanging around with Adam, some of his friends, and a couple of girls from my old school in the year below me for a couple of weeks now. All we did was sit in a large group on the grass in the castle grounds, enjoying the hot sunny weather and talk about all sorts of things. I never wanted to be a burden and talk about my depression with everyone because I didn't want to bring anyone down, but at least I felt less depressed when I was with my friends. I found out that Adam was into me but I was not into him enough to get into a relationship. If I'm honest I still felt unsure about having a relationship with a guy due to the judgement and discrimination I could have faced. I had been messaging a girl named "Stacy" from the year below me at school and she had also been hanging out with us in the group. "Stacy" is the name I'm using to represent this person as she doesn't want her real name used in this book. I was fully aware that Stacy suffered from depression and had also self-harmed. One of the first times

I ever met her properly in person was when I bumped into her after school, when I was meeting Charlotte, and I had noticed some cuts on her wrist. I was really enjoying her company and I found myself gravitating towards her when we were all together. She was so easy to get on with and she understood the pain I was in. After hanging out in a group all day, pretending to be really happy, we messaged each other online where we could really open up about our emotional struggles. It was the first time I had truly connected with someone who was as genuinely depressed as I was. And my god did I find her attractive.

I was falling for Stacy pretty fast and didn't waste much time in telling her about how I felt about her. We decided to meet up alone for once so we could talk more openly rather than have our friends around to distract us. It was that afternoon, beneath a large tree in the Rochester castle grounds, that I told her that I liked her. I felt so nervous telling her that I liked her because I wanted her to like me back so badly. She was perfect for me for so many reasons. She was caring, open, funny, interesting and beautiful, she was everything I wanted in a woman, not to mention she wouldn't judge me for self-harming and she understood what depression felt like. But to top it off, like me, she wanted to commit suicide. I was still in a state of mind where I wanted to kill myself but I was afraid and I didn't want to do it alone if possible. I didn't want to get caught like I had before and I believed that dying with Stacy would be the "perfect" ending. Once I told her that I liked her she responded with, "I like you too." Despite all the shit I had been through she made me feel happy with that response and over the next few days we labelled ourselves an official couple.

Our relationship got off to a flying start and it felt so right. When we were together we spoke so openly about everything and I felt comfortable in sharing my deepest darkest thoughts with her. I didn't feel ashamed or awkward when she saw fresh cuts on my body and neither did I when I saw similar afflictions on her skin. We had an understanding where we wouldn't talk about it if we didn't want to and we wouldn't force the other person to open up if they didn't want to.

When we weren't together we spoke on the telephone and through social media as often as possible, even though we had spent time together during the day.

The summer holidays were more bearable now that I had someone to share it with that I was falling in love with. She was able to hold off my feelings of depression and anxiety when I was with her, like she was some kind of miracle drug. It's a shame I couldn't be with her overnight as that was the time when the depression came back. Without Stacy I had no distractions that were good enough to hold the urge to cut myself at bay. I remember one evening feeling lonely without her and my mind was producing thoughts that reminded me that life wasn't worth living. Even though I was in a great relationship suicide was still a priority of mine, especially now that Stacy had confessed that she wanted to commit it with me. From time to time, in the days where we were both feeling down about life, we discussed how we would commit suicide with each other. I had the idea of slashing our wrists, and evening slashing each other's at night time were we would be found dead. I also had the idea of taking an overdose as it could be less painful. As sick and as strange as it may sound It felt pleasing to discuss suicide with the person I was in love with, it was like we were writing the "happy" ending to our own love story.

There was one occasion where Stacy and I performed self-harm together, not on each other but on ourselves whist in each other's company. On this particular occasion our emotions were all over the place, we were happy to be in each other's company but our individual circumstances and our pasts were having a dark influence over us to the point where we wanted to harm together. I can't explain this without it sounding sadistic or psychotic but harming together brought about a strange sense of relief and satisfaction that I had only experienced when I was on the edge of the shopping centre roof that one time. I only ask that you, the reader, stay open minded about this and that you must remember that people in seriously negative states of mind do things that *ordinary people* may deem "crazy" or "wrong". Please don't judge me for engaging in this activity.
The two of us removed some of our clothes and went to the bathroom, as any spilt blood could be easily cleaned from a lino floor rather than a carpet, with our blades. My Dad's bathroom was very small, there was only room for a bath, toilet and sink, all three of which were squeezed together closely. Stacy sat upon the toilet whilst I stood in the bath. I felt a moment of hesitation, like I always did just before making the first cut, but with Stacy there I didn't feel I could just stand there and think about it for ten minutes like I did when I self-harmed alone. I looked over into Stacy's beautiful brown eyes and smiled as I made the first cut on my left wrist. The endorphins kicked in quickly, along with a sick sense of satisfaction. I hate to say this but at the time cutting myself never felt so

satisfying. Self-harm is so personal so sharing it with the girl I loved made it somewhat special, if you can call it that. I'm not attempting to romanticise self-harm, it was just different to self-harming alone. Stacy took her blade to her right leg and made a gash about the size of my thumb, I had never seen someone self-harm in front of me, especially someone that I loved, so I didn't know how to react. I just watched to see what would happen. Of course blood came pouring from the wound down her beautiful pale and skinny leg. I asked her if she was okay, even though she smiled at me whilst performing the seriously large incision. As much as I was "enjoying" this I couldn't help but feel concerned for her so checking on her seemed appropriate.

I made a few more cuts on my wrist, leg and torso. I wanted to feel the pain like never before, I wanted Stacy to see me as I was at my most vulnerable, but most of all I wanted to share that part of myself, and of herself, that had never been shared before. I know it sounds weird but I felt closer to her than I had before. I knew she was the one for me.

When the cutting was done we cleaned ourselves and the bathroom up as one drop of blood left behind would have been enough for my Dad to interrogate me. There was plenty of blood but it wasn't hard to clean, most of mine was in the bath tub so I got rid of that by turning on the shower.

There's no doubt our fresh wounds were sore after that unusual experience. We both wore skinny jeans and they didn't help, the material would rub the cuts with every movement you made. I put my black arm warmers on as usual to the hide the cuts on my wrists. As I mentioned before, this was always uncomfortable but that's the price you have to pay if you want to self-harm in secret and be left alone.

Over the next month or so my life continued to be fairly consistent. Stacy had started Sixth Form at the beginning of September and during the day times, whilst my Dad was at work, I'd sit in his flat, alone, planning the end of my life and self-harm from time to time. I'd then go and meet with Stacy as often as possible after Sixth Form and when I wasn't working at the restaurant. I continued to see the rest of my family in small doses on weekends. Stacy got to meet my family and I got to meet some of hers, fortunately we were hits with our respective partner's families. I still received the bog-standard insults from people when out and about on my own, or, with Stacy as I still dressed alternatively. I even received a few insults from a girl when the two of us went to Camden market in London. I

was impressed with Stacy after she give this girl some verbal abuse in return though. I always thought Stacy was brave compared to me.
In general, all was going well to be honest, it wasn't enough to make my depression or anxiety go away but it was enough for us to stop wanting to kill ourselves. Stacy was the first person of the last two years who had convinced me to stay alive, and, with her by my side I felt like I could take on my challenges with a little more confidence and positivity than usual. You could say things were looking up a little for me.

Chapter 9 – Another Experience in a Mental Health Ward

Not long after Stacy had convinced me, through her sweet and gentle love, that we should continue to live and enjoy our lives together I found myself still struggling to cope with the pressures and challenges of my life. Although I was madly in love, which helped bring light into my darkness, Stacy was in Sixth form and I had became envious. I was envious because I had ruined my chances of getting any qualifications through the normal education route that teenagers took. In my eyes she was enjoying herself and had a plan all figured out but I didn't and my lack of a goal was bringing me down again. I didn't mention this to Stacy because I knew she had her mental and emotional demons to fight and our relationship was going smoothly. I didn't want to be the first one to make a complaint or put a negative element into the positive chemistry the two of us had. I did what I always did, I took it out on myself and told no one about it, I let my skin do the talking for me.

Even though I was living with my Dad I stayed over at my Nan's house more often than not. Her house was nearer to work and the Sixth Form that Stacy attended during the week, not to mention that my Nan cooked for me and drove me around places when I needed a lift. I felt like I had more privacy at my Nan's house unlike my Dad's place, my Nan had a bed for me in the conservatory which meant I could self-harm without worrying about someone interrupting me in the night. Don't get me wrong, I found something that resembled happiness in my relationship with Stacy but the rest of my life and the thoughts that I had about it were hard to cope with. I wanted to live for Stacy's sake but it was stressing me out trying to hold myself together for her when everything else was making me feel unbalanced. I believed I was a disappointment to my family, I believed I wasn't liked at work, I believed that I was losing some of my oldest friends, I believed that world was out to get me and I believed I was a nobody that was going nowhere. I was self-harming almost daily to cope with the pressure that weighed on me and it got to a point where the disappointment got me in a vicious cycle. I needed to self-harm to cope but I was ashamed at how much I cut myself and how much I depended on it, which made me want to do it even more. I felt more out of control than ever.

One evening, when my Nan had gone to bed, I waited for her to fall asleep so I could do some damage to myself. I had been going through the same routine each night for the past week or so. I would spend the day thinking about harming myself, see or speak with Stacy once she had finished Sixth Form, I went to work a couple of evenings in the week and then I'd let my Grandparents, or Dad depending on where I was sleeping that night, get ready for bed whilst I prepared to cut myself. The routine I had for self-harming was the same as it had been for the past year or so and tonight was no different; I would get a small amount of toilet roll from the bathroom to soak up any blood that spilt, get out my hidden razor blades, give them a quick sanitising wash and then get my iPod and start listening to a playlist I made that was filled with about fifty or so songs that I listened to motivate me into hurting myself. If you have been in this position you will know what I'm talking about. It's not as easy as you think for someone to just instantly pick up a sharp object and take it to your skin, sometimes you need a little encouragement in order to get yourself in the right frame of mind for self-harm. I didn't always need the music but it gave me time to reflect upon the day, or past experiences or anything else that was making me feel depressed. I usually listened to a couple of songs before harming but I never listened to music whilst harming. This was because I didn't want to get caught and having headphones in my ears didn't allow for me to hear anyone potentially walking in on me mutilating myself. That wasn't a risk I was prepared to take. During the week I had also thought about returning to the mental health ward where I stayed previously in July. I didn't feel very safe and I believed that going back there was a good idea for several reasons; firstly I would be watched over, secondly I still felt the world was out to get me so being in there would keep me protected and thirdly I needed a break from the pressures in my life. Okay, it was boring, pretty depressing and I was cut off from my normal life but at the time I thought going back to an isolated ward was a good idea.

So on this particular evening I pushed my regular self-harm routine a little further to see if I could get back to the ward. I knew I couldn't just call up and go in like last time as I hadn't made an attempt on my life or anything of that sort. Instead I took some pills, more than I was supposed to according to the manufacturer's label, as well as slicing my wrists and thighs. I remember being extremely angry with myself and the way things had been going of late so I put more force than usual into cutting. It hurt, it fucking hurt, more than usual, and very rarely did I cry whilst self-harming but this time I had to let the tears flood. I was scared about going back to the ward and equally scared about my future and my current circumstances, it was too much for me to hold in. And of course the disappointment for what I was doing to myself made it worse. Like I said earlier, self-harm is a vicious cycle.
Once the damage had been done I walked out to the hallway, whilst bleeding out and only wearing a pair of boxer shorts, got in a foetal position on the carpet and called out for my Nan to wake up. My Nan had never seen me like this and I felt awful for putting her through it but she was calm as a cucumber when she emerged from her room. She asked me what was going on and why I had done this to myself, I asked her to call the crisis team at the hospital and see if I could go back.
At first the phone call didn't go the way I had planned, I was explaining that I felt like killing myself and that I wasn't safe to be at home or anywhere else and that I needed to be in the ward but they refused. It wasn't until I kept on at them, whilst sobbing down the phone, and explained I had taken a small overdose did they agree to see me. Although I was in physical pain from the cutting I felt a little relieved from an emotional standpoint.

I was taken to the hospital and went to the same waiting that I sat in the last time I ended up on the ward. I couldn't here that noise that I heard last time, you know, the one that sounded like a patient screaming for help? I wondered if it was something to do with the air conditioning but I was too afraid to ask about "the noises". They might have thought I seemed crazier than I already felt.
I sat there with my Nan in this empty room, waiting to be seen, whilst in complete silence. The wooden chairs in the waiting room were very uncomfortable and my wrists and thighs were stinging which meant I couldn't sit very still. The waiting and the pain, not to mention the depression and anxiety, was unbearable and I kept fidgeting my legs and hands. I kept thinking to myself, "Please let me on the ward." I had no

idea what I was going to do if I went back home after this, I didn't have a plan for that.
After what seemed like hours of silence and discomfort two male mental health nurses came and asked me to follow them into a room, the same room I was assessed in last time I went on the ward. I sat opposite them at a desk with some closed blinds to my right. One of the nurses seemed grumpy and lacked a smile but the smaller nurse appear a little friendlier. I sat there hunched slightly over the desk with my hands on my knees, a dry throat and a face that resembled the lowest amount of enthusiasm you could possibly imagine, I had a typical depressed face. They asked me the usual questions, like, "What's wrong?" "Why have you done this to yourself?" "Do you want to kill yourself?" I gave them honest answers and told them that I wanted to kill myself because I felt like I was a piece of shit that had no future, that I was verbally and physically attacked and that, to some extent, that I enjoyed hurting myself. I also mentioned that I planned on committing suicide in the not too distant future.
They finished their questioning and let me sit outside in the waiting room with my Nan, I did nothing but hold my head in my hands and stare at the floor feeling completely empty. A little time passed and then the nurses came out and told us that I would be omitted onto the ward. Once again I felt relieved and fearful, but, at least this time I knew what to expect. At least I thought I did.
I said goodbye and goodnight to my Nan and then made way for the ward. I followed the two nurses up to the ward and it was just as ominous as it was the first time, maybe more this time. I felt like a freak, a mess, mental, crazy and miserable all at once. Going in the second time lead me to believe, at the time, that I was a true "mental person" with nothing to offer the world except pain and frustration. Even with the lights on in the corridors it felt like darkness surrounded me in the hospital, I guess the dead silence made me feel that way as I dragged my feet across the floor. I wanted to be in the ward but at the same time I didn't, if that makes any sense? I wanted the safety but I knew the isolation, and being around the other patients, was going to be depressing.
I reached the ward and it was as silent as a graveyard, all the patients were sleeping in their dorms and rooms. I was escorted to a room with five other occupied beds in it and all I could think was, "Shit, I'm going to have to share this room with some other crazy people."

Upon my first morning I realised two things; one, was that I was in the ward next to the one I was in last time, the one that appeared to have patients with more *severe* mental health problems, and two, I quickly learned that my routines would be the same as last time. Though there were some subtle differences that made this stay a little more "challenging". After breakfast I was taken to one side and shown my belongings, which I had to hand over the night before when I entered the ward. The nurse, opened my bag I went through it with me to remove items such as belts and cables, you could guess as to why this was couldn't you? I didn't argue about it either, if I wanted my phone to be charged I just had to ask for them to do so in the secured room. Another difference of course was the patients, though there were a handful that I recognised before. Michael, the little old man who got whacked on the head was on my ward, so was Ronald, the jolly old fella. A few women from last time where here also. I wondered if they had been here all this time in the two months since my last admission.

In the first couple of days there I struggled to sleep, my depression and anxiety had a tendency to do this to me, no matter how tired I was. Sometimes I used self-harm as a way of getting to sleep. I know that sounds ridiculous but when you're addicted to self-harm, and I mean *really* addicted, to the point where you're doing it almost every day, you can end up self-harming even though you've had a half-decent day, or nothing bad has happened in particular, just so you can get some sleep. The endorphins that get released when you hurt yourself feel so relieving and they calm you down. If you can't sleep because things are on your mind you can get the urge to hurt yourself just so you can feel the endorphin release in order to relax and fall asleep. The problem was that I couldn't do this on the ward. I was pleased that they moved me to my own room during my first whole day there but the room was dull and blunt, with nothing sharp for me to cut myself on, so I struggled to sleep. When you've got depression and anxiety and you're struggling to sleep it's very stressful. All the shit you hate and fear just sits in your consciousness for what feels like hours. You keep tossing and turning trying to get comfortable and calm. But your mind doesn't rest, it keeps giving you things to think about, things that you can't do anything about because you're trying to sleep. No amount of self-talk can get you to calm down and relax because talking to yourself is just another way of stimulating your mind.

Nothing worth mentioning happened on day two either, I just felt lonely and miserable like always, with the exception of a visit from Stacy. She had the power to lift my spirits at least, but they dropped again when she had to go home, which left me feeling empty and guilty for putting myself in the ward. But when day three came things started to get a little different. I was due a meeting with the doctor, or psychiatrist, or something. With the amount of different professionals I had seen in the past two years I struggled to keep up with who's who. Anyway, during my assessment I was asked the usual questions that I had been asked a million times before. I told them the usual, "blah blah I want to die blah," feelings that I had and the fact I was struggling to sleep each night. But on top of that I came to a realisation the day before that I could hear voices, or more specifically one voice, telling me to damage myself and telling me things that made me feel shit about my own existence. It seemed sensible to share this with the person assessing me.

I didn't fully understand whether this voice was a product of my highly stimulated imagination or if it was the result of my current mental and emotional state. Up until I shared it with the psychiatrist I had not given much thought to the inner voice that was telling me to harm myself because I thought it was merely my conscience gone bad. It was hard for me to make sense of what this voice was so sharing it with a mental health professional was quite difficult.

I described the voice as a bad influence that tried to get me to hurt myself more often that I'd usually desire and that when it spoke I had an image in my head of a heart monitor, the screen with the line that goes up and down in line with your heart rate, and the moving line was neon green but went fuzzy and wild when the voice spoke to me. Don't ask question why this was, I have never tried to under it to this day, all I know is that being in a dark place mentally has the power to create unusual thoughts, mental habits and things you don't want to comprehend.

The more I spoke of this voice the more I began to accept them as real whereas before they seemed to be something in my mind's background. It actually started to make me feel more anxious the more I spoke about it because I never wanted to be one of those people who struggled so badly with mental health problems that they had to depend on help for the rest of their lives, or worse, be thrown in a padded cell for being a threat to society. Fortunately the psychiatrist put my mind to rest and explained that there was medication for such things; they were called anti-psychotic drugs, which seemed like a heavy hitting name to me, and that they would help put the voices at bay until I gained more control over my mentality. Initially I thought, "Great, more pills" but it couldn't get any worse could it? Oh, and I was prescribed some sleeping pills too. The anti-

psychotic drug is known as Quetiapine and the sleeping drug was Zopiclone
That evening at nine o'clock, which was medication time, we all lined up like cattle for our pills. When I got to the dispensary booth I was provided with the usual anti-depressants and then I got my two new pills. I swallowed them without hesitation and went back to my room to feel sorry for myself and stare into space whilst questioning my entire life. I laid on my bed listening to my iPod, the same sad and angry songs that I always listened to, but it wasn't long before I started to feel really spaced out. Ten or so minutes into taking my new pills I felt high as a kite and I couldn't move or mentally function like I would normally. I felt light, slow and sludgy. I could talk to myself internally and give a running commentary on my slow bodily movements but I felt like my mind and my body were two completely separate entities. I didn't like it either as I felt very out of control and touch with reality. Being in a confined environment like the hospital made me feel uncomfortable already and this wasn't helping. Not that it mattered as I fell asleep almost instantly shortly after experiencing that bizarre high.

The next morning, day four of my imprisonment, I was woken up for breakfast and I felt like shit. As a depressed teenager I generally woke with the feeling of resentment and grogginess but this was something else. The pills I took the night before must have left me feeling like this. I struggled to get dressed and make my way to the canteen area as my mind was so hazy. It was like a hangover but without the nausea. When eating breakfast I felt like everything around me was happening without me being there, it was like I was a ghost that was spectating the world going by. Everything seemed so far away and I wasn't making any effort to talk to anyone, not in this state. I wanted to get through the day and avoid people as much as possible. Whilst chewing my cereal I still felt groggy and spacious to an extent but I managed to conclude that this was just my body getting used to the new medication.
After breakfast was over I was made to line up for my pills again. I was expecting just to take anti-depressants but my new anti-psychotic drug appeared to be a twice a day thing as well. I didn't say anything to the person administering the pills and I went along with it. Down went the pills.

Back in my room I was getting ready to take a shower when I was hit with more dizziness. Somehow I was even more spacious than before. I then

stumbled over to my bed and closed my eyes. This new drug I was on was unbelievably strong.
The next thing I know I'm being woken up by a member of staff asking me to come down for occupational therapy. They left the room for me to get myself together but I couldn't. My head was spinning and I could barely stand without feeling like I was drunk or something. This new anti-psychotic pill was doing a number on me and no matter how hard I tried to be consciously aware I was losing control. I was beginning to hate these pills very quickly. I told the mental health staff that I wouldn't be attending occupational therapy due to this medication screwing around with me. In the afternoon I was a lot fresher after another nap and found it relatively easy to walk to the canteen for lunch. I even made small talk with some of the other patients which was a big step for me.
The rest of the day didn't hold much excitement or anything out of the ordinary though; I sat in my room, doing nothing, I had visitors in the afternoon, ate dinner, etc. Most of my stay was extremely tedious as you might have gathered. There was one exception though, that afternoon I heard shouting and banging at the entrance to the ward, my room was only twenty or so feet away from the front door so I heard everything. I poked my head out to see a woman in her thirties, Jane, whom had been a patient here on both of my visits to the ward, trying to kick down and pull the front door open with every ounce of energy she had. I had seen people lose their cool but this was a new level that I hadn't seen before. Two members of staff were trying to calm her down but she wasn't willing to give up. She kept shouting, "Let me out, I want to see my kids!" I watched for a few moments before hiding back in my room. I put my headphones in and let the music drown out the shouting. I couldn't help but feel sorry for her. It was bad enough being in here, let alone being trapped in here and not being able to see your own children.

On day five I arose from another deep sleep induced by the new pills. I felt a little clearer in the head this time, my body must have started to get used to it perhaps, so going for breakfast was unchallenging for once. As usual I ate breakfast and took my pills. I was a little slower and reluctant to take the anti-psychotic pill this time and the dispensing nurse noticed this so they made me open my mouth to prove I had swallowed it. I'm not sure if the hesitation was a symptom caused by anxiety or if I just didn't want to fall asleep again. I walked back to my room dreading what was about to come next; dizziness and losing control. Right on schedule, I fell asleep and was eventually awoken by staff to get ready for occupational

therapy. In my hazy state I pushed myself to get ready and I took deep breaths to try and wake up. I liked occupational therapy as it was something normal for me to engage in and I needed to feel normal for once.
I walked down to occupational therapy, keeping myself to myself as always, with a little dizziness still keeping me from operating at full capacity. On the way down I noticed a woman, possibly in her late twenties up to mid-thirties, I was crap at guessing peoples' ages, whom had be omitted to the next door mental health ward the day before. I only noticed her because she was dressed a little more alternatively, like myself, and I was feeling lonely and desperate for someone to talk to that wasn't going to judge me. I was grateful that I could text and call Stacy, my Mum and my other loved ones outside of the ward but I couldn't do that all day and visiting times were so limited.
Down in the occupational therapy room I sat on the sofa watching the other patients get involved in activities when this woman, whom I previously mentioned, came over to sit near me and then started talking to me. I was nervous about approaching any of the patients for a chat because I still hadn't sussed them out to know if they were dangerous or easy to talk to. The woman, who introduced herself as Ayesha, was very open about her own problems and was interested in what I had to say about my own challenges. I wasn't used to opening up to people I had just met, with the exception of mental health professionals, but I sensed that she wasn't going to start judging me for the way that I was. We actually got on pretty well, talking about all sorts of things from our emotional difficulties to our personal interests. It was nice to make a friend during my stay there and I didn't feel alone so much now. It was a shame she was in the ward next to me, as all the patients from the separate wards could only converse during the time of occupational therapy, otherwise I could have had a friend to talk to pretty much all day.

On the way back from occupational therapy I was feeling better about myself for making proper conversation with one of the other patients, instead of the usual "good morning" and other meaningless curtsies. Also on the way back I was met with an awkward situation; to get to my ward we were made to walk through the mental health ward adjacent to mine. As we were walking back one of the female patients, skinny and in her late fifties, was staring at me as I walked towards her through the corridor. She was just standing there with empty gaze waiting for me and as I went to walk past her she grabbed me by the shoulders and stared

into my eyes for a few seconds. I had one of my headphones in my right ear, listening to my music, and this woman verbally insisted that my headphones belong to her. I was stunned by the her actions, I practically froze up. She grabbed them until some of the staff managed to pull them out of her grasp. I quickly walked away as it honestly frightened me. She looked harmless but you never know with people who are unstable.
As I got into my ward the same woman who tried to rob my headphones was being wrestled and dragged, whilst she was screaming and trying to fight off the nurses, into the isolation room.
The isolation room was next to the main shower room and I had a little peak in there earlier that week. It was the room you'd expect to have padded walls in but it wasn't quite what I imagined. Inside was just a mattress, no bed frame, no padded walls, no straight jacket or anything else. The walls looked tougher than the plasterboard walls in my room and the door was certainly heavier; it had a small round window in it like you see on ships.
This woman was not co-operating in the slightest and for a woman of her size and age she was putting up a good fight against two considerably larger male nurses. I was impressed by her determination if anything. But it wasn't her day and she was eventually dragged into the isolation room. The two male nurses slammed the door shut and stood there catching their breath whilst the angry woman screamed the room down. A few of the patients from my ward and I watched from the living area whilst this went on. Trust me, this sort of thing livens up your day when you're stuck in a place like a mental health ward. I could hear her calming down after five minutes of trying to kick the door down and scream like her life depended on it. Once the screaming stopped she tried to convince the nurses that she needed the toilet, as there wasn't one in the isolation room, but the male nurses were smarter than that and they kept her in there. They were all trying to negotiate some sort of deal and at that point I was bored enough to go back to my room for another lonely night.

Day six in the fun house and I was feeling optimistic about the upcoming weekend. The day before I had spoken with Stacy about going to Camden Market on the Saturday if I was allowed out. I had been allowed out during my first visit so it was possible that I could go out this time too. Some of the mental health staff had hinted that I might be able to go out if the doctor, or psychiatrist, forgive my lack of remembering the correct title, was able to give me the all clear. I had a meeting after lunch time scheduled with the "doctor" so I knew I could make that request then.

Until then I just needed to be on my best behaviour and come across as positive as possible so that I could improve my chances of some freedom and sanity.
Before my meeting I went down to occupational therapy to enjoy the company of Ayesha and this time I was going to make more effort to make conversation with other patients, the ones that looked friendly to me at least. Whilst down in occupational therapy, or OT as it was known, I got talking to two other people; Jane, the woman who wasn't allowed to see her kids, and a tall man named Carl. Carl was hard to miss, not only was he pretty tall but most of his skin was damaged. After gaining his trust through deep and thorough conversation I had the confidence to ask him what had happened him and why was he admitted. He seemed very gentle and had a soft warm voice, a kind of gentle giant if you will, and in his calm voice he explained that he had previously set himself on fire. Once he said that it made sense as to why his skin, including the skin on over fifty percent of his head, looked rough and white in comparison to the rest of his brown skin. When he told me that he'd set himself on fire I didn't bother to ask why, even though I really wanted to know, but I had a feeling the answer was either going to haunt me or not make sense to me. I couldn't help but feel for this guy, he seemed so psychologically together by the way he was talking to me, and if he didn't have scars all over him you'd think he was just a regular guy. But that's what mental health problems are to the untrained eye; invisible.

Later that day I went into my assessment meeting in high hopes thinking that I was going to get granted day leave on the Saturday. I did my best to convince the man talking to me that I was feeling much better, that the medication was helping keep the voices at bay, that I didn't want to die any more, even though that was bullshit and I tried to hold a sincere smile on my face the whole time. Once his questions had been answered by me I asked him if I could be granted a day leave on the upcoming Saturday. My hopes were shot down pretty quickly as if I didn't matter to him, which I probably didn't. All day I had been super excited and experiencing an emotional high but now I felt like the remains of a burst balloon. I stormed out of the assessment room with my fists clenched and walked right into my room, which was almost next door, and slammed the door shut and screamed into my pillow. It didn't take me long to calm down and start turning that anger into sadness. I had a habit of turning angry and frustrating feelings into sad and depressive thoughts. I laid on my bed starting at the ceiling thinking, "What the fuck am I going to say to Stacy?"

and the usual, “My life is so fucking shit, I can’t wait to die.” I know this seems dramatic for being told “No” but when you’re experiencing depression and other emotional difficulties this is just another nail in the coffin to make you feel like shit.
That afternoon I had the dreaded phone call conversation where I had to give the bad news to Stacy. I wasn’t looking forward to letting her down, she was so special to me and I already felt like a fuck up so this wasn’t exactly going to be easy to deal with. Like the awesome girlfriend she was she took the bad news pretty well and she expressed her interest in me getting out of the hospital as soon as possible. As much as I was pleased to talk to her on the phone and hear her soft and loving voice it made me really miss life on the outside. At that point I realised how much I truly hated being isolated on the mental ward. It’s such a lonely place to be in, no matter how many patients and staff are in there with you it’s still lonely as hell, and, the paradox is that you don’t really want to speak with anyone in there most of the time because you just want to dwell in your own emotions and thoughts. With that I was starting to feel a strong urge to self-harm, it had been over five days since I last cut. Being given false hope of seeing the outside world was really driving me mad. When you’re trapped in a mental health ward it’s hard to find something to actually do some damage to yourself with. Like I mentioned before they take the stuff from you that could hurt yourself with and blunt objects are no good as they tend to make a lot of noise. In frustration I punched myself in the jaw and side of my face a few times. I wanted to cut so badly and feel that release. I was desperate to cut myself!

I sat on the edge of my bed looking around at what I possessions I had, all of which were not sharp, but, I realised had a CD case from a copied album I made that was of little value to me. “What if I just snap that appropriately and use the sharp edge of the plastic?” I anxiously thought to myself. It seemed like it could work and that it would be easy to pull off. It wasn’t going to be as sharp as the razor blades I normally used but it would have to do on this occasion.
I grabbed the CD case and wrapped a hoodie around it to suppress the snapping sound. I had my door closed but I didn’t want to take any chances of someone hearing the plastic breaking. With a little effort the case broke into a few pieces and one part was ideal for cutting. I picked up the slightly jagged and triangle shaped piece of plastic slowly and my heart started racing. It felt like Christmas day when you unwrap that one present you wanted above all others.

I did have a second of hesitation because I was scared that cutting myself might keep me in there longer, I knew hiding it wasn't going to be easy, but that thought didn't last long. With a held breath I put the sharp piece of plastic to my wrist and pulled it across my skin.
Nothing happened, other than a very thin layer of broken surface skin. Using this plastic to make me bleed wasn't going to be as easy as I thought. So with all of my effort concentrated and the plastic blade firmly gripped I yanked it down and across simultaneously. This time blood was visible.
It was a different kind of pain this time though, probably due to the fact I had to apply some pressure on the blade, which wasn't usually the case. I did it again and again until I had between twenty and thirty superficial, but satisfying, cuts across my left wrist. The pain was good, to me at least, and I felt a little more stable and calm, I use the term "stable" very loosely here. Although my need for pain had been met I was still lonely so I stepped outside my room and sat at the door until a member of staff notice what I had done. I never did anything like that before, I usually tried to hide self-harm from adults but the loneliness was unbearable. Any form of company or attention would have been good.
A member of staff did see me on their routine hourly patient check and came to my needs. They cleaned my wrist up and put a bandage around it to cover the cuts. Just like everyone else they asked me why I did it and just like nearly every other response I said, "I don't know", and I left it at that. I thought doing this might keep me on the ward a little longer but I didn't really care how long I was in there any more, I was just miserable, lonely and wanted to die.

Day seven was just like any other day on the ward but I wanted to try a little harder at making conversation with some of the other patients this time round. Occupational therapy was really good that day as several of us, including Jane, Ayesha and Karl, plus others, sat round the sofa having a good old natter. Every now and then I kept visualising the group of us as normal people rather than patients locked up against their will. The conversation was fun and almost meaningful, it was the most normal I had felt throughout my stay and that means a lot to a person with emotional and mental issues.
I took to Jane quite a bit that day and she was on my ward so I had the privilege of talking with her for the rest of the day. Jane was almost twice my age but incredibly easy to talk to. When the evening came we sat together in the living room space sharing our stories of struggle and

general "getting to know you" things. Her story and the things she had experienced shocked me and left me feeling emotionally sick, more so than I already was. I'm going to share with you what she told me, but, it's not for the faint hearted so please skip the next two paragraphs if you feel uneasy or emotionally fragile at this point.

She started out by explaining that she ran away from home when she was in her early teen years as she was heavily mistreated at home. When she ran away she eventually ended up staying at this couple's house, who were complete strangers, and was there for a while. The couple were not quite the caring couple you'd assume them to be. Jane shared with me that the couple, who were sexually open, agreed that the man should impregnate Jane. By this time I was on the edge of my seat and the rest of the world around me faded into nothing but what came next disgusted me more than anything else I've ever heard. She said that once her baby was born the couple wanted to give it a ceremony, to which Jane got excited about.
Imagine this now; you're a messed up teen who has ran away from home, knows very little of the world, has been kindly taken in by a seemingly nice couple and then got pregnant, pretty heavy stuff right? So a nice ceremony for your new baby sounds cute and harmless doesn't it? At this point I wish to mention that the baby was born at their house and wasn't registered. Jane got her baby all dressed up and looking both smart and cute for this ceremony, but, it turned out the ceremony was actually a ritual. I won't go into too much detail but I will say that Jane had the unfortunate experience, to say the least, of watching her baby be sacrificed.

At this point I could have exploded with tears of rage. I didn't ask any questions out of respect and out of fear of any more shocking experiences. There was a very short pause before Jane continued with her life story and the pause was so short it was almost as if she had become comfortably numb with the experience she had just shared with me.
Jane had two daughters and told me about her partnership with the father of her kids, which only continued to make me clench my fist and feel depressed at the same time. She described the father as violent and perverse. I'll leave you to make up in your own mind what that could mean.
I noticed that Jane had some really deep and heavy scaring across both of her wrists, way more damage had been done to her wrists in comparison

to mine. The healing of her older scars had raised the skin quite a bit where there was so many scars. I really felt for her and the situation she was in. The story she shared with me, the one you have just read, seems so tragic it's almost hard to believe but if you, the reader, could have seen the state of her wrists and got to have known Jane you would deem the story true just like I do.

On a slighter lighter note Jane, whom I felt very close to now, made me laugh by telling me that when she got bored of being in the mental ward she sometimes called up help lines and told them that the plug sockets were trying to talk to her. If this was true I would have felt concerned but as it was just a joke and needed a laugh, after a few serious stories, this made me giggle. She then proceeded to get out her mobile phone and call one right away to show me. I had to cover my mouth where I was trying not to laugh. Jane got through to someone and told them she could her the plug sockets and light switches speaking to her. The person on the other end of the phone must have heard me cackle because they hung up pretty quickly. Trust me, stupid little things like that are highly amusing when you're depressed and stuck in a mental ward not knowing when you're getting out.

Let us skip now to day nine of my stay, because day eight was pretty standard in terms of events. I had an important meeting and assessment scheduled just after lunch and I was told my Mum, my Dad and my Step Dad Nigel would be attending. I was feeling extremely anxious and apprehensive about this meeting because I knew that *feelings* would be spoken about a lot and that was never easy to discuss with family around. I spent all morning in my room panicking then staring at the walls, or the floor, whilst trying to hold myself together. I had only just gotten in the habit over the last few days of staying out of my room and talking to people but it was like I had forgotten about that and instead I isolated myself.
When the meeting was about to initiate I was escorted from my room to the meeting room at the end of the corridor where there was a small cluster of people. Nigel, my Mum, my Dad, a mental health nurse from the ward, my psychotherapist and another doctor were sitting in a circle waiting for me. It was quiet and all eyes were on me as I walked in slowly and anxiously. My heart began to race, my stomach dropped and my hands were shaking; bloody anxiety!

I went over to the only empty chair in the room and sat very cautiously waiting for someone to start talking. But when they talking started I zoned out to reflect upon my past and anticipate my future again. I had a habit of doing this when people spoke about things I didn't want to hear.
I managed to control my attention for a while whilst my psychotherapist started talking. I took a liking to her a little while ago as I had been seeing her for a few months and she didn't hold back. She was rightly firm and very clever, it's a shame because she always managed to make me feel good during my past sessions but the effects never lasted for more than a day. She was pretty firm with all of my parents, which was sadly satisfying for me. I say sadly satisfying because I couldn't believe I had to get this far into my struggles for my parents to listen and be more understanding, I know they tried but it was never enough for me.
As things were being explained to my parents I sat there with a dry mouth trying to hold back tears from feeling like a failure within my family. Not to mention that I felt awkward as they were getting a "telling off", if you will, for the way they had misunderstood and dealt with me. To be honest I was more worried about what Nigel was thinking as he and I never saw eye to eye on a lot of matters, I didn't want him to hate me, or himself, after this meeting was over.

After everybody's feelings, thoughts and professional opinions had been vocalised it was agreed that I would be leaving the next day and I would return to living with my Dad at his flat. I can tell you now that I left that meeting with the most mixed emotions I had ever had. On one hand it was great that I could finally get the freedom I wanted, see Stacy, my friends and get back to a normal routine but on the other had I was afraid of the world and a large part of me was suggesting that my life would get worse. But still, at least my parents seemed to have more empathy and a clearer understanding of me.

Chapter 10 – A Cut too Far

Fast forward now to December that year, 2007, and things were about to take a turn for the worst. Life after the mental ward visit was pretty much the same in terms of events and experiences, but at least my family were better equipped to understand my needs.
I was still living at my Dad's, some of the time, and at other times I stayed at Stacy's home that was round the corner from the restaurant I previously worked at. I had quit there not long after my stay at the

hospital but I struggled to live without income and I got bored of being at my Dad's place with little to do in the evenings. In relation to my depression and self-harm I was still in deep and the cutting hadn't stopped. I was at my best when spending time with Stacy but she was still studying during the day and I couldn't be with her as much as I wanted to be. I was still fifty-fifty about wanting to live. It becomes so frustrating when the good parts of life and the bad parts keep trying to cancel each other out because you can never have peace of mind. At least when you know what you want to do you have something to go by. But it was my relationship that was currently having the upper hand so living was my current choice.

In the time that Stacy and I were together I learnt that she was prone to health problems, I'm speaking in terms of physical health now, and just before Christmas she feel more ill than I had seen before. I don't find it necessary to share the details or symptoms of her illness but it was bad enough that it put her in hospital.
I remember going to the hospital with Stacy and her Mum Jeannie late one evening whilst feeling extremely concerned. I had never had much experience with hospitals for myself or loved ones when it came to physical illnesses so this was beginning to bring on some anxieties for me. I felt helpless enough as it was but this was becoming increasingly hard to deal with. I was in love so much and I hated seeing her so ill and in discomfort. By the end of her assessment from the doctor she was omitted into the hospital for further observations and tests, then Jeannie took me home that night back to their home where I slept in Stacy's bed; alone.
Two days later and she was still in there whilst they were trying to get to the bottom of it all, which left me feeling highly anxious about her recovery and our future. Now, you could say I had nothing to worry about and that everything was going to be ok, and you could be right, but to a teenager that suffers with depression and anxiety, who's also madly in love, this was freaking me out and bringing me down really low. My thoughts were unbearable to deal with so much so that I felt like the suicidal part of me was taking over. It was scaring me how low I felt.
I was with my Dad at the time and I begged him to take me to the hospital so I could be seen by someone as my psychotherapist was not available at short notice. He spoke to someone and they told us we could go to the emergency room for someone to talk to me as soon as possible.

Then the urges to harm myself started to generate inside me. But it wasn't an urge like I had before, it was more intense than usual, like, crazy intense. Sorry for my poor use of English but that's all I can describe it as. My Dad got himself ready and called a taxi whilst I dived into my bag to find my razor blades. I wasn't exactly thinking constructively or cleverly, in fact I had no idea what I was thinking, but the urges were taking control of me. It's really hard to convey what was going through my mind and what I was feeling at that moment, the best I can come up with is that it felt like something was possessing me to do some serious damage to my body and that I had to go along with it.
I grab my blades and hid them across several places; one in my phone's battery compartment, because that was a thing at the time, one in the battery compartment of my portable games console, one in my arm warmer and the rest of the pack in my pocket. I wanted to be sure that I could really inflict some harm on myself. Again, please don't ask why I was doing this, it just felt like something I needed to do.

On the journey to the hospital I could think about only two things; Stacy and how I was going to hurt myself. I thought it would be a good idea to go to the A&E bathroom whilst waiting to be seen and then cut my wrists and bleed out till someone found me. I had noticed a week or so before hand that since performing deeper cuts on myself with razor blades I could see the layer of bluey purple tissue, I think that's what is was, beneath my skin. When being a fool and trying to open my wounds I could see where some of my veins were so I thought today would be the day that I adventure into cutting deeper than usual. The idea frightened and excited me.

We arrived at the hospital and entered A&E where the receptionist gave us the lovely news that it could be up to a four hours before I was seen, "Fucking great!" I thought. I turned around to scope out the environment that I'd be spending the next several hours in. I could see plenty of people sitting round waiting with the look of boredom and frustration on their faces, I was going to fit in just fine. My Dad and I took a seat where he proceeded to read a newspaper and I pulled out my iPod. I put on my "Slit Wrist" playlist, the playlist that I usually listened to before performing self-harm so I could psyche myself up. As the songs played through my head phones I kept on thinking about how my plan was going to be executed. The idea of bleeding out in the bathroom still seemed reasonable so I wandered off to have a good look in the men's bathroom.

I walked in and it was empty, which was good as I wanted to take a good look round before actually doing anything. The floor was a clean but faded beige colour, the walls were pretty much the same and there were a couple of cubicles next to the sinks on the left. It was a basic public restroom but it seemed clinically clean enough to perform some incisions of my own.
I left with a slightly clearer picture in my head as to how this was all going to go down. I figured that all I had to do was wait an hour or so and then sit on the toilet and cut deep into my wrist. Bingo.
For the mean time I just had to sit and wait for the pre-assessment to be over and then I could get on with it.
After forty five minutes my name was called out for the initial assessment. I walked over to the room near the bathroom where the doctor was due to asses me. I sat down with the doctor, who seemed fed up with how his day was going, based his tone of voice, and he asked me some questions. I received the same questions I had had a million times before from the various people who had assessed me and it was becoming annoying having to explain myself an express my same thoughts over and over again to different people, but, this time I just kept it simple and told him I wanted to die. I thought maybe keeping it simple might actually get me some help a little quicker.
Once the pre-assessment was over I walked back to my seat and did my best to act like I wasn't going to do anything. A little time went by and I ventured off to the bathroom again to try and motivate myself. I sat on the toilet and pulled out a blade from my pocket. That strange overwhelming feeling I got when I was about to cut started to circulate through my body. I held the blade tightly between my finger and thumb, with my heart beating fast, but I couldn't do it. It just didn't feel right. I had never cut in a public place before. I took a deep breath and slowly put the razor blade back in its packet whilst flushing the toilet to make it seem like I had used it. On the way out I took a quick look at myself in the mirror to compose myself. I didn't want my Dad to pick up any signs that I was feeling uneasy and about to self-harm; I wasn't always good at hiding things when I was at my lowest.
Two hours of sitting in the waiting room had gone by now and I was struggling to hold myself together. As the rest of the world faded out my imagination was presenting my consciousness with images of me bleeding out on the hospital floor. This was all I could think about right now, because I wanted it to happen. I had fantasised about suicide so much since my last attempt and I was feeling more up for it than ever.

Everything that was keeping me alive was fading from my mind and all of my depressive memories and my current anxieties were taking over. My mind was full of the things that made me want to die.

"Scott Shrubsole," a nurse politely shouted from across the other side of the room. The A&E waiting room had two adjoining areas that you went to once you was ready to be seen; the mild injuries area and the critical injuries area. Although I didn't have a physical injury, the nurse took me to the critical injuries area. My Dad was told to wait in his seat whilst they spoke to me. As I followed the nurse I felt pretty gutted that I didn't use my waiting time wisely to go to the bathroom and cut myself. "What the fuck am I doing with myself?" I thought frustratedly. The nurse took me over to a private cubical that was sectioned off by a curtain and told me to sit and wait on the bed that was in the cubicle. I looked around at this small area to examine the available medical equipment, as there was little else I could do. The was a pot to urinate in, a box of medical gloves, a breathing mask and canister, a roll of disposable clothes and the obligatory, yet ironic, yellow sharps box.
Five or so minutes passed and my previous idea was still flowing through my mind. "What if I do it here?" I wondered. Once again the rest of the world disappeared whilst I only foresaw myself bleeding out in this little curtain railed cubicle. On the other side of the curtain were lots of doctors, nurses and patients making plenty of noise but that all drowned out whilst I reached for the razor blades in my pocket. For a few minutes my life was silent. It was so surreal; it was like the only things that existed were me and the blades. I took a brand new blade from its box and unwrapped it from its paper packaging. I held it in the palm of my right hand for a moment to examine its shiny surface, and when I did images of my arms bleeding flashed in my mind.

The time had come for the fantasising to end and for the desire to become reality. In my hazy state of mind I brought the blade to my left wrist and gently pressed it against my skin. I held my breath, as the world around me continued to remain silent, and pulled down.
I looked down at the blood whilst feeling high off the endorphins my body was producing. I sat there with a satisfied feeling and a messed up grin on my face that only people like myself could understand. But I wasn't going to stop there. I made a few more incisions on my left wrist, and these cuts were carried out more aggressively than usual so the blood was flowing a little faster and thicker than usual. I looked at my left arm and thought,

"This isn't enough," and I started on my right wrist. I hated cutting my right arm because I was no good with my left hand but at that moment I didn't give a shit about anything. I cut the word "Fail" into the upper area of my right wrist, which was quite clear, and then made two horizontal cuts at the lower part of my wrist, just below my palm, and one diagonal cut through them.
There was blood on the hospital floor, on the bed and on me. Plenty of adrenaline was flowing through me and I was beginning to shake and rock back and forth. I still had no perception of the outer world beyond this cubicle I was in. I was listening to my iPod the whole time this was going on and I found myself listening to particular songs that matched the intense emotions I was feeling. Then it dawned on me; I looked down at the largest of the cuts on my left wrist and then I used a disposable towel to try and soak up some of the blood for a few seconds. I soaked up enough blood to just about see a vein beyond the bluey purple tissue. I sat back down, very very slowly, and held the razor to the wound. My muscles started to lock up, my stomach felt sick and I had one last image flash in my mind; it was an image of doctors and nurses picking my body off of the floor. With the blade held slightly within the wound, ready to cut the vein, I closed my eyes and paused. Then I pulled down, hard.

As I opened my eyes my perception of the world was not only silent but now everything seemed to have slowed right down. I felt disorientated, dizzy and light headed. In my slow state I looked down at where I made the last cut and I watched the blood pour out like a carton of cherry juice being squeezed. It was pouring out quicker than any amount of blood I had lost before, in fact I was used to blood dripping or trickling out, not pouring out. A puddle of blood was forming on the floor next to my left foot, I could see splashes of blood on the edges of my shoe. I watched a little more blood flow until I started to feel sick and too dizzy to stand. I was numb all over, I just couldn't feel myself and I was losing grip on my reality. "Finally, this is it," I thought.

My mind was blank, I could hear nothing, I could see nothing and I could feeling nothing. I was only barely aware that I existed. But then fear stuck me and I regained a clearer consciousness. I looked down at my wrist again and the amount of blood I had lost was shocking to see. This fear of dying was changing my perception enough to want to live, but it didn't feel like me. It was more of an instinctive state, and in my instinctive state

I pulled the cubicle curtain out of the way and slowly dragged my feet enough to walk out and shout for help. "Help me please"! I pleaded. My survival instinct that had given me enough strength to seek help started to fade away and I was becoming so dizzy I could barely stand. I dropped to my knees and in my barely conscious state I felt a couple of sets of hands lift me up on the bed and another hand pull my left wrist above my head. I was purely a spectator who could barely make sense of what was happening. I can just about remember hearing the words from a male nurse, "He's brought blades in here with him." The dizziness was getting so bad, due to the blood loss, and I thought I was going to be throw up.
The male nurses managed to get the blood loss under control and wrap my wrists up in bandages as I sat on the bed all limp and lifeless. I felt so emotionally distraught and with my consciousness starting to become clearer I was also feeling shameful. I hated my life but I hated myself for doing these crazy things to myself, yet the paradox was that I felt like I needed to punish myself and that I needed the pain to feel in control of myself. If you self-harm you probably know what I mean.
The pain from my wrists were very uncomfortable now that the endorphins and adrenaline were starting to wear off and instead they were replaced with the feelings of guilt and self-pity. "Why do I do this to myself?" I asked myself with my lip quivering. My eyes started to well up and form tears that dripped onto the floor next to the blood from my wrists.
I wanted to zone out and disappear from this situation but the male nurses escorted me to an observation ward that was just round the corner. I was told to sit and wait on the bed until a psychiatrist could see me, which was potentially hours away.

Half an hour later, at about three in the afternoon, my Dad was escorted to my bedside when he said, "I walked past a pool of blood back there and I should have known it was yours." He had a genuine look of care and concern on his face, the look that I didn't see too often but it was enough to feel make feel loved at least. My Dad, as you'd expect, started questioning me as to my actions but I wasn't in the mood to talk about it. I was half in pain, physically, and half wanting to shut out the world. I made it clear to him that if he wanted me to talk I wouldn't talk about what I had just done to myself. I still hated talking about my feelings and when I felt distressed I could never talk to my family about it. I laid on the bed, on

my left side, with both wrists rested in front of me to avoid as much discomfort as possible, because my wrists fucking hurt.
I continued to lay there in this weird foetal position with my eyes aimed at the wall opposite me, but really I was staring into space playing the image in my head over and over again of the cuts I made in the cubicle. Watching the vein start to empty in my head was oddly satisfying, probably because anything relating to suicide excited me.
Forty five minutes after my Dad found me my Mum arrived and she was all over the place; asking me questions in a panicking and concerned state. I didn't want to talk to my Mum about this either. Over two years into my depression and being asked the same questions over and over gets unbelievably tiring. "Why do you feel like this?" "Why do you do this?" Sometimes I just wanted to scream, "Leave me the fuck alone!" But I could never say that to my own Mum, I generally had more respect for her than that. Plus I felt guilty to some degree.

Hours and hours went by and the small observation ward, which only had four beds and patients, was starting to make me feel claustrophobic. My Mum and Dad were still trying to talk to me, the other patients were moaning and the nurses kept walking in and out. I wanted silence but the noises were constant and driving me crazy; the footsteps, the complaining, the chatter, the beeping, the ticking of the clock, all I wanted was to disappear from this small room into nothing.

Around ten in the evening a nurse came to look at my wrist. She unwrapped the bandage slowly and I was looking in anticipation to see what my wounds looked like, especially the deepest one. Just thinking about it now, whilst writing this book, makes me feel tingly and uncomfortable in the stomach and on my left wrist where I now have very visible scars. When the bandage and the patch that was used to bung the wound were removed I could finally see what I had done to myself. It wasn't pretty, at all; I had never done anything this destructive to my skin before. The wound was about as wide as my thumb, if not a little wider, and was roughly two inches in length. The worst part was I could see a layer of myself that I wasn't meant to see; I had cut beyond skin and looking at it made me feel sick again. Guts and gore was easy to handle but it wasn't like what you see in horror movies, oh no, the real thing on your own body is very different. I looked away and let the nurse get on with it. With her gentle hands she dabbed a sanitising fluid in the wounds, which stung like a bitch, and proceeded to put butterfly stitches on a few of my wounds. I acted like it wasn't hurting but it did, my wrists were so sore and so was my head. Losing blood and crying isn't exactly a soothing experience for the body. But now I was ready to see the psychiatrist, after waiting for over eight hours.

Let's just say that night ended with me on a new anti-depressant, a new therapist and a slightly new outlook on myself. I wasn't quite ready to die just yet. Cutting a vein and experiencing that level of trauma, although self-inflicted, taught me to appreciate my life and my circumstances a little more than usual.

I was done for the night, putting myself through that left me exhausted. Time for bed and tomorrow will be a new challenge to face.

Chapter 11 – Bad Decisions and a Serious Suicide Attempt

It had been months, ten to be precise, since I had slashed my wrists whilst inside the A&E department of my local hospital. A lot had happened since then, mainly the stability of my relationship with Stacy. Admittedly I had been a selfish dick behind her back, kissing other girls, and a guy, and thinking I could get away with it. I wasn't bored or not in love with Stacy but the pressure of life, the depression and the anxieties, had a weird way of influencing me to to do things that I shouldn't, including being selfish and not using my brain prior to making decisions. I'm not in anyway trying to justify my behaviour, I know I fucked up. I didn't like what I did, I was never proud of what I did and it disgusted me that I was following in my father's footsteps by making out with people that I wasn't in a relationship with. I didn't have the balls to tell Stacy, I could barely admit my mistakes to myself, let alone admit them to the person I actually loved. You might be reading this thinking, "How could you have loved her if you were kissing other people?" You're right to ask that, and even I would ask that now, but depression, anxiety and feeling suicidal leads you to indulging in things that the body desires that give a "quick fix". For some it's food, gambling, alcohol or drugs but for me it was self-harm and sexual pleasure, even if that meant kissing someone that I shouldn't have. I'd just like to clarify again that I'm not blaming my mental health issues at the time for my actions, I still had, and will always have, the power to make my own decisions. I was just in a habit of making bad ones when I was on an emotional low or high.

So I put myself in a position where I was riddled with guilt for my actions over the last few months, June till October to be exact, which lead me to cutting myself. I felt so stupid for thinking I was smart enough to have my cake and eat it. Stacy had been nothing but amazing to me even when I didn't deserve it. She forgave me once where I pushed her on the arm to try and getting her fighting spirits up, a stupid decision on my behalf again, and I didn't deserve her forgiveness. That ended up in an argument, her in tears and she locked herself in the bathroom to escape me. I had a real problem with understanding how to understand and empathise with people sometimes.
Not only did I kiss some people, show a lack of empathy, get into stupid arguments but I was also controlling. Being of the alternative fashion I really tried to get Stacy to wear certain things even when she just wanted to dress normally. Stacy liked alternative fashion but had to be in the mood to want to wear certain items of clothing where as I went all out all the time. As much as Stacy was perfect to me I still tried to get her to wear clothes that she didn't just so I could be satisfied for whatever reason. I also got her to try things in the bedroom that she didn't want to from time to time, another reasons for me being branded a "dick".
It's not easy to share these things with you, because no one wants to come across a fool, failure or a dick to anyone, especially an audience of people like yourselves but I'd like to believe you can, like I did, forgive my mistakes as a stupid teenager and continue reading my story.

October of 2008 was the month that Stacy and I split up. It wasn't due to the fact that I had gone behind her back and been inappropriate with other people. It was more of a mutual agreement that came out of an argument one Sunday morning before I had work. We were at her house and we decided to end it after arguing about something I can't even remember. I was probably being an unsympathetic, arrogant or ignorant, which I had a tendency to be when I wasn't focused on putting myself in the other person's shoes. We ended it together out of disagreement and tension, which then turned into tears and cuddles in her bathroom. I felt relieved for about five minutes after leaving her house, as I would no longer be putting her through any more shit, until I got to work and that's when I started to regret it. Although I did the typical male thing and tried to hide it from my work colleagues. I wished I had just worked through the argument instead of taking the easy option of breaking up.

In the few weeks that followed our break up I was a mess with a bit of hope. Stacy and I were still in contact, I even still slept over hers a few times. I was still clinging on to her hoping that she would take me back, which I made clear to her that I would if she was prepare to have me back. But that hope was shattered one morning when I woke up in her bed and she told me that it wasn't a good idea me staying there when she wasn't honestly wanting to get back with me. I walked out of her house that morning in shame, disappointment and with my eyes staring at the ground.

It took me a little while to accept my fuck ups and the fact Stacy wasn't going to take me back no matter what I did but I was still struggling to feel happy. Hearing the words, "I don't want to get back with you", for the first time practically broke me in two. Although, for my past behaviours, I knew I deserved to feel miserable. The one person who made me feel a little secure, a little special and even a little happy had now gone. When I wasn't at work I laid on my bed most of the time thinking about how much I hated myself and my life more than ever. Stacy gave me hope for a future but now that was in ruins. I couldn't see a way out of my depression so I was right back where I started; believing that I was too much of a failure to make anything good happen and that I would be miserable forever. And I *still* had no idea what I wanted to do with my life. Everything from my past, such as the bullying and my parents arguing, kept playing in my imagination over and over again too. With all this on my mind practically 24/7 I resorted to self-harming daily. Since cutting myself in A&E I had managed to self-harm far less than I did before because Stacy ignited this flame of life within me. But now I had lost her thanks to my stupid actions and decisions, so all I wanted was pain. I wanted to feel the pain that I had once caused.

In December of that year I decided I would kill myself, and, I would do it right. Before I felt like I had nothing to lose, in relation to my previous attempts, but now I genuinely felt like I had nothing to lose. Stacy was everything to me and I couldn't live without her by my side. I had enough of crying into my pillow at night, I had enough of feeling lost and I had enough of cutting myself to escape the emotional pain I was in. I couldn't stand feeling like a black sheep in my family, I couldn't stand feeling worthless and I couldn't stand waking up without a purpose any more. So I made a plan, which was a little more concrete and serious than the ridiculous plans I had of jumping from a roof in previous years. I was still on heavy anti-psychotic and anti-depressant medication and judging by the fact that the anti-psychotic medication knocked me out for over an hour each time I took them I guessed they would kill me if I took enough. I had missed taking some of my pills on purpose and I ordered repeat prescriptions earlier than required so I could ready up a bulk of pills for my suicide. Some nights I even did some research on the internet as to the best suicide methods, not that I found much as most websites tried to discourage you. When that wasn't doing anything for me I just looked at people's photos of self-harm on social media and watched films that involved suicide. Like self-harm I felt that I had to get into the "zone" in order to carry out a suicide attempt. Believe it or not I managed to hide all of this from my friends and family, none of them had any idea I what I was planning. I acted like everything was fine during the day, like my break up meant nothing to me. I played the part of a "happy teenager" really well, it helped that I could drive by this point as I was able to go out and meet friends and show them all how "happy" I was.

Then came the evening of my planned suicide. It was the middle of December, I was living with my Nan, who had gone to bed, and I was all alone. I slept in the conservatory at my Nan's house, which gave me some much needed privacy. All eighteen year olds need privacy right? Who doesn't?
Anyway tonight was the night and I was up for dying. It was fairly dark in my room, all I had was the light of the bedside lamp to illuminate the conservatory, and I suppose it was the right lighting for the mood I was in. In my wooden bedside cabinet were my pills, including all the extra pills I had saved or randomly gathered from here and there, which were now stored in a jiffy bag. I made myself a glass of water from the kitchen sink, a large glass at that. I sat on the rug next to my bed for a few minutes to think about what I was about to do. I felt so dead inside I didn't even panic or have an increased heart rate any more. I put on my pyjamas, sat up onto my bed and stared into nothing for a few moments. Everything around me seemed to just disappear into silence but the depressing, traumatic and displeasing events of my past took their turns in reaching my consciousness until they all had my attention for one last time. But it was Stacy's face that came into my mind's eye the most. I missed her so badly that it brought tears to my eyes once again.
I wiped the tears away and proceeded to empty the packets of pills onto my lap. I had no idea how much it would take so I emptied at least fifty pills, most of which were from my box of anti-psychotics. Before I took the

first pill I could feel the same disturbed feeling I got when I self-harmed but it was more intense and I felt like my burdens were about to be completely lifted. With my left hand I picked up a pill and placed it on my tongue, then I sipped enough water to wash it down. "Ok I can do this," I hesitantly thought. My heart started beating a lot fast at this point. Then I picked up a few more pills and gulped them down with some water. I started to pick up the pace and shove as many pills in my mouth as I could realistically swallow. I could taste some of them going down the back of my throat. They tasted horrible, almost making me gag.

Before I new it I had swallowed over fifty high dosage prescription only anti-psychotic pills. I didn't feel humorous but I smiled to myself in that sick way like I did when I self-harmed sometimes. I quickly hid my empty pill packets under my bed then slowly climbed under the covers. I didn't feel the least bit scared to be honest as I believed this was the end of me. I smiled to myself one last time before switching the light off. "Goodbye shit life," I thought.

Chapter 12 – Awake

At the time I hadn't planned on getting this far with my life. I hadn't planned on waking up to see another day. The earliest memory I have of regaining consciousness was when I could just make out that My mum was trying to feed me yogurt and Nigel rubbing his hand on my forehead. I was only conscious for a few seconds and then I feel back into deep sleep. The next time I woke up I was more aware of what had happened. I had no idea what day it was or what time it was but what I could make out was my family standing there in front of me. My Mum, Nigel, Dad and my Nan were there standing in front of my hospital bed. Once I saw them all and slowly realised where I was I just let myself cry my eyes out. I was too weak and so ashamed to hold back the tears this time, even though I hated crying in front of people. I wasn't just ashamed that my family had found me in this predicament, I was also ashamed that I had failed in my undertaking.

I still didn't want to be alive. I was too weak and could barely talk but in my head I was screaming in emotional pain. "Fucking kill me!" was a re-occurring phrase that flew around in my head. The more conscious I became the more aware I was of the damage I had caused myself. It was a

good thing I could barely move otherwise I'd probably had rolled over onto one of the cannulas I had in each arm. That's right, I was hooked up to two drips. I then suddenly felt the need to take a piss and it was at that moment I realised I had a catheter installed. I had to use it but it felt so uncomfortable and unnatural. Even now recalling it into my memory leaves my downstairs region feeling awkward, let's put it this way; I hope you never have to have one. I started to notice some beeping too. I looked to my right and I could see some monitors that had had cables coming out of them and they were connected to my chest. I couldn't believe it had come to this. I couldn't believe I had got here, I didn't want to be here, I was supposed to have died!
The first day I regained consciousness was one of the most depressing days of my life. Dealing with the fact I had tubes and cables attached to me was one thing but having my family surround me was another. I had already cried enough once my consciousness was regained but as the day went on I felt more and more depressed. The family were all constantly talking to me and giving me love but I just wanted to die. In the times that they left me to get some rest I stared at the heart monitor for hours and visualised my heart rate drop until it flat lined. I wanted it to happen so badly but it never did. I ended up falling asleep instead.

It was lonely being in the critical care unit, but I wasn't as lonely as I was uncomfortable. The cannulas in my arms were sore, I tried so badly to keep my arms straight but I had to move them from time to time, usually when I needed to urinate into the catheter tube. That required some skill in itself. The sounds of my machine, and the sounds of the other three machines in the room was driving me crazy. Beep beep, beep beep and beep beep over and over again. I didn't want to talk to the nurses, nor did I want to talk to the other patients, so all I could listen to was beeping. I did speak to myself in my head a lot, not only to drown out the sound of the beeping but because I couldn't self-harm so saying unpleasant things to myself and thinking unpleasant thoughts was the best I had.
I was in the critical care unit for several days and every day was pretty much the same except I made a little more progress in my recovery each day. I didn't want to though. I never properly prayed before but now I was wishing for death. I wanted my heart monitor to flat line or for some sort of organ failure. I would have been grateful for any kind of death. Even when my family came to visit me I had no change of heart, I just wanted to die. Being stuck in a bed was helping my physical recovery but it didn't help with my mental recovery. The frustration, pain and anger made me

want to die more than ever. Being in hospital made me often think back to the previous year where I had cut my vein in the A&E department, when I did it made me wonder if I could do something like that now, but as much as I fantasised about it I never felt like I had enough energy to pull it off. Instead I asked myself, "Why do I deserve this and when am I going to die?"

During my several days in the critical care unit my Mum visited me the most out of my family. To be honest she did bring me comfort, as much as I wanted to die. She told me, which still surprises and shocks me to this day when I think about it, that I was found on the floor by my Nan the morning after I had taken the overdose. Apparently I was cold, stiff and completely unresponsive. What shocked me the most was that she said when the paramedics arrived to take me into the ambulance I was trying to fight them off and that they struggled to get me on a stretcher. I couldn't believe my ears as I had absolutely no recollection of these events what so ever. I tried to imagine what that looked like but the idea of an unconscious person fighting off paramedics seemed ridiculous. But it happened my Mum assured me. But there was something else my Mum shared with me, and at the time I thought nothing of it, but it still plays over in my head regularly today. She told me that the doctor said, "Scott's body threw itself out of the bed during the night, if that had not happened he would have died if another hour had passed." The only thing that saved me was the fact I rolled out of bed and on to the floor, which never happened in the hundreds of times I had slept in that bed. If I had stayed in that bed for another hour my Nan would have found me and presumed I was still asleep, thus I would have passed away. When I was first told this I wished I had stayed in the bed, but today I have a very different outlook; I'm glad my rolled onto the floor.

Once I regained my strength in the critical care unit, which made a week feel like a year, I was able to go down to another ward where I could be for the rest of my recovery. I was feeling a bit more "lively", excuse the pun, by this point and I bothered to make friends with some of the other patients. I went out with them for a roll up each day, which was surprising as I could have just ran off at any point to try and commit suicide again. I came back from a cigarette once to find my Mum waiting for me, she wasn't very pleased and told me that the doctors suggested I might have a permanently weakened heart and liver, it didn't put me off smoking as I couldn't have given a shit about my life at the time.

My friend Richard came up to visit me, who was the first and only friend that visited me whilst in hospital this time round, and it was hard to approach a conversation with him. When he came to my bedside I threw my arms around him and held a firm grip. I found it easier to be more emotionally inviting towards my friends when going through my struggles and this was no exception. But Richard had a stern look on his face, like a mixture of frustration and sorrow. It was understandable, he had been a great friend of mine for the last seven years, regardless of what we had been through before, and I nearly ended our friendship. "I cried when I heard what had happened," was the first thing I remember him saying to me. That hit me hard, I felt like I had been a bad friend for doing what I had done but at the same I didn't regret it, I only regretted waking up.

After about a week of recovering in the second ward since the overdose I was given the all clear that I could return to the outside world. I had gotten used to being in hospital; the routine of the meals and health checks, the comfort of not having anything to worry about; love, money or bullies. The other patients I made friends with made the experience a lot less lonely to. Part of me didn't want to go back to reality. In a weird way I associated that particular hospital admission with death and that's what I found more comforting than anything. Death, suicide to be exact, was what I wanted and coming away from it brought back the things in my head that made me depressed and anxious.
I remember walking out of the entrance to the hospital with my Mum, it was a dark and wet December evening. It had been raining all day and it was cold, my body usually had a strong internal system for staying hot but on this occasion I was still a little weak, so I wrapped myself in many layers whilst sitting in the back of my Mum's car. I sat in the back looking out the window feeling a bit sick, I hadn't taken any of my meds since overdosing and I was starting to go all delirious from the withdrawal symptoms. I wasn't allowed to take my meds, for obvious reasons, but I really wanted them. When I missed taking my anti-psychotic I had a tendency to start thinking really twisted thoughts; in the self-harm sense, and feeling really nauseas.
When I arrived back home at my Nan's it didn't feel as relieving as it did when returning from the mental health ward the previous year. This time I was very apprehensive and had no desire to return to reality. I continued to have a little voice echo in the back of my mind that repeated, "I wish I was dead," every few minutes or so. But I had some unfinished business to attend to that had the potential to inspire my last shot at redemption.

Walking up the garden path to my Nan's front door I thought it was a good idea to risk calling Stacy one last time. For one stupid reason or another I hoped that my suicide attempt had made her realise how much she meant to me and how far I was willing to go in order to secure her love for me. Yeah I know, what an idiot I was right?
Let me clear this up; I didn't attempt suicide purely to get her affection, that fact she rejected me after all my efforts had worn thin was just the final blow to my struggles.
As soon as I got in the house I made way to my room, which was so surreal as it was the last place I was conscious whilst in the house, only to find my fold up bed folded up where the paramedics had tried to make space to keep me alive. The room was more untidy than I remember leaving it.
I got tidied up, even though I felt so weak and drained, and then got onto my bed so I could relax and make a call to Stacy. I laid down on my bed with a little shaking in my hands and with my heart pumping fast. I was in high hopes of a good phone conversation and everything working out, it was the most optimistic I had been in a while. As the phone began to ring I could feel my stomach jumping around in anticipation, "She'll take me back, won't she?" I kept worrying. The ringing seemed to go on forever. "Oh please pick and take me back," I pleaded in my head.

Stacy eventually picked up the phone and we spoke briefly about my recent suicidal episode. I don't need to divulge in what was said, instead let me skip to the outcome; she didn't want to get back with me, which left me in the same emotional state I was just before I swallowed a fistful of pills. On the phone to her I tried to translate my feelings into words but the intensity in which I loved her wasn't conveyed well enough, in my opinion, and no matter what I said it wasn't enough for her to take me back. When the phone call ended I laid there, staring at the ceiling, wishing the earth would open up and swallow me whole. I wanted to disappear forever. All that went through my mind was, "I need to stock up on pills again, my life is over."
In later years I accepted and understood why she didn't take me back at the time; I was suicidal, I kissed other people, we argued and I was controlling. I didn't provide her with the love and care that I should have. But at the time I didn't accept my mistakes, some of them I didn't even recognise. All I cared about was being in her arms again, to be kissed and loved by her because she made me feel alive. She made me want to walk

this earth. Without her I was a mess, a nobody, a failure of a human being.

Chapter 13 – Depressed and Trying to Survive

In the first few days back at my Nan's house I was all over the place. For once the physical discomfort I was in overthrew the mental and emotional torment I usually wrestled with. I hadn't taken any of my meds for nearly two weeks, I think, as I was made to let my body naturally flush out as much of the substances as possible. On the first full day of being home I was due a home visit from my new care co-ordinator, whom I had seen a few times leading up to the overdose. But I felt rough, the withdrawal from my crazy pills was making my stomach feel twisted, almost similar to when you've not eaten all day but much worse. I was lying in bed waiting for Mark, my care co-ordinator, to arrive when I felt the nausea and disorientation manifest. I knew my body needed the pills because the nausea and disorientation always kicked in when it had been over twenty four hours without the medication. I rolled around on the bed trying to distract my mind from wondering into darker places but the nausea was getting to me. I ran out my room and into the garden to throw up. That's when Mark arrived and came out to find me in that state. Not the most flattering welcome.

He let me return to my room to recover whilst he caught up with my Nan and Mum, who had come get the low down on my care. I really wanted to talk to Mark but it was hard to even stand up without feeling like I needed to vomit. But in the end I managed to drag myself out to him, hunched over like I had back problems, and ask him some questions.

The first thing I had to know was when I could start taking my pills again as the withdrawal was unbearable. It was far worse than most of the experiences I had been through during my depressive state. He could see how much distress I was in, which may have worked in my favour as he informed me that I could start taking them that evening. "Thank fuck for that," I sarcastically thought. I did have to promise that I wouldn't overdose though, which wasn't any easy decision to make. Honestly speaking I said I wouldn't but there was still a large part of that was lying just so I could get my hands on the medication. I was prepared to do literally anything to get my hands on my meds.

The rest of what Mark and I discussed was mostly about returning to work and my ongoing care with him. I was lucky that Mark was still able to work with me. I know that some people aren't able to work with people when they attempt suicide. I looked forward to my appointments with him as I could really let go and lay my cards out on the table without feeling like I had done wrong.

Now, let me tell you about Mark and my sessions with him. Over the next two or so years I went to visit Mark for an hour either every week or two weeks, depending on how miserable or stressed I was, at a hospital in Rochester. My last therapist, the lady who took little bullshit, was ok to work with but Mark was on a whole new level that I was highly receptive to. He also didn't take any bullshit and had something to throw back at me every time I shared my experiences, troubles or feelings with him. I admired what he said to me and the way in which he engaged with me. My last therapist came across a little angry and frustrated when I opened up to her but Mark was great with his body language and the tone in which in spoke to me. Unlike previous therapy sessions I was actually excited to visit Mark, not just to unload my problems on to him but also to receive his words of wisdom. There was something comforting about Mark that made me to want to listen to him instead of just ignoring his advice, like I had done with previous therapists.
Every week or two I'd drive up to the hospital, in my shitty little Fiat Punto mark one, and struggle to find a parking spot, walk into the front of the hospital, sign in and go in and sit in the waiting room. The waiting room was right next to the reception so I could hear what everyone was in for. It was surprisingly rare for me to be waiting with other patients, and only on one occasion can I remember someone waiting to visit a mental health therapist. I usually sat there in silence, trying not to make eye contact with anyone who walked by, on the same arm chair each time listening to sad songs on my iPod whilst trying to remember all of the things I wanted to talk about with Mark.
My first few sessions, after the overdose, were not as constructive as they could have been though. Because, deep down, I still wanted to die so generally I went around in circles with Mark about my feelings and problems. We would sit in a room, no bigger than an average bedroom, that had a couple of chairs, a coffee table and a box of tissues and then my emotions would come flooding out for Mark to try and defend himself, which he did without even breaking a sweat. But I'd still try and find problems with his solutions. Since battling with depression, consciously or unconsciously, I seemed to make extensive effort to find

reasons as to why the advice I was being given wouldn't work, no matter how much respect I had for the person trying to help me.
We mostly spoke about my suicide attempt in my earlier sessions with him. Wasting no time at all Mark asked the question that everyone had been asking me, "Why did you do it?" With the amount of times people asked me that I had trouble trying to keep up with the truth, nearly everyone got a slightly different answer each time I tried to answer. But I had no trouble at all being straight to the point with Mark. "I feel like I'm a failure, the love of my life won't take me back, I struggle to get along with my parents and people bully me for being myself," that was as black and white as I could have possibly been. For the next two years Mark and practically covered these topics every week.

Early 2009, after a couple of months of therapy with Mark, I had come to accept not having Stacy in my life. It wasn't an easy thing to accept either, I had self-harmed quite a bit in the months leading up to the acceptance. Although dying was on my wish list I hadn't planned for it any time soon so self-harm was the way that I vented my darkest thoughts. With this acceptance I forced myself to get back in the dating game. I believed that moving on would help me fill the void inside of me that was once filled with Stacy's love, though in my heart I didn't want anyone but her. I did what most young people did and went online to look for someone to start talking to, and every Monday I went out to the local alternative club to try some "real-life" luck.
It felt unnatural at first to try and meet someone new, partly because I didn't want anyone but Stacy and partly because I had lower confidence than before. I'm still unsure whether my lowered confidence was due to being rejected by Stacy or if it was down to how low I had sunk into depression. But to my surprise I managed to make out with a couple girls at the club and eventually meet someone online who became my girlfriend shortly after.

Falling for another person that wasn't Stacy felt exceedingly surreal. I had never hidden any of my dark, weird or unpleasant feelings and experiences from Stacy, I didn't need to because she was so open minded and caring, and I knew I would struggle to keep my past, and present, from my new partner. Trying to kill myself wasn't even that long ago, in the grand scheme of things, and on top of that I self-harmed and suffered with depression and anxiety. Not exactly the easiest things to hide from a new partner. I got lucky though, my new girlfriend was quite accepting of

my problems, which helped her open up about her personal problems. I didn't open up about everything all at once though, I only shared with her what I deemed to be sensible and relative. I couldn't exactly say, "Yeah I tried to kill myself after my ex wouldn't take me back because I was an asshole."
But unlike Stacy I didn't exactly feel comfortable in sharing my current deepest and darkest feelings with my latest partner. On several occasions I self-harmed and then showed up at her house the next day just for her to question me and heavily urge me to call her when I felt down. But I couldn't, I wasn't afraid to show my new partner my fresh cuts but I wasn't prepared to talk to her when I was feeling shit enough to cut myself. I had only ever done that with Stacy, I was so close to her that I struggled to share that unstable part of me with anyone else.
So my new girlfriend had to put up with my cutting every now and then. But the tables turned a few times when I came round her place to find that she had also cut. I felt like a hypocrite when I told her contact me in the time of need. But that's just one of the things about people who self-harm, it's very difficult to turn to someone for help when you're at the point of "no-return". Once you've made your mind up to cut yourself, or whatever method you use, you forget about calling out for support. It's usually after the deed is done do you turn to people for help, by then it's too late though.

I think that relationship lasted about sixth months tops. The relationship, from my side at least, was quite enjoyable but after a while I became discontent. There wasn't anything wrong with her at all, but deep down I still had strong feelings for Stacy and dragging that feeling about with me in a relationship was too much to bare. In the later part of my relationship it was weighing me down, like I was carrying the burdens of the entire human race, so I had to end it. I felt pretty guilty for that too, I timed it so badly it's almost comical. She was drunk and throwing up all over her front porch when I called it quits with her. I know, I was a dick right? Again, not proud of myself at all. At the time I absolutely was a dick, but you make poor decisions when there's chaos in your mind and when your heart and head are out of sync. At least now I could go on without dragging anyone down with me.

Throughout 2009 I did very little to make progress with my mental health. Every day and week become a monotonous blur of repeating actions. I still lived with my Nan. I worked every day of the week except Thursdays at the same restaurant I had been at for three years. During the day times I either played video games or surfed the web. I saw family every once in a while, and I gave them the impression that I was doing well; they bought it too. I met with friends for drinks every Monday and got pretty drunk at the club. And I still had no aim or purpose. I know this sound like the typical life of a nineteen year old but all I was doing was living on autopilot. I never woke up and thought, "I'm so happy to be alive and my life is so awesome!" I was lucky that even on a few occasions I woke up and felt alright. In addition to that I was still taking my anti-depressants and anti-psychotics day in day out, which after a while made me believe I was going to be on them forever.

But the thing that did change was that I was a better actor than before. I mentioned in the previous paragraph that I managed to convince my family that I was alright, I also managed to convince my friends, my work colleagues and pretty much everyone that I came into contact with. I attended all of my therapy sessions with Mark, I managed to leave no evidence of any blood loss wherever I ended up cutting, I made effort to meet with people instead of blowing them off, I took my pills every day and I made extensive effort to look happier. And I didn't dress as alternatively as before, I stopped wearing eye-liner and was a more open to colours other than black. I was trying to put on the most convincing show on earth, and it worked. It was pretty fucking difficult to pull off though, especially when it came to hiding cuts and any blood I had lost. I got caught out so many times before when my Nan, or Mum years before, had found blood in my bed, on the carpet, on my clothes and even on paper towels in the bathroom bin. I had to up my game when it came to an eye for detail, it was like covering up a crime scene. My blades were never found either. I kept up the act long enough to make everyone around me believe that I had stopped self-harming and that I wanted to live. I could have received an award for my acting that year.
"But where did you vent your thoughts and feelings?" you might ask. Putting on a front like that wasn't easy and even self-harming wasn't enough to express my struggles with failure and a lack of purpose. I worked so hard to hide my darkness from people that I had cut off my chances to talk to anyone about it, except my therapist Mark. But I didn't have access to him outside of my sessions so I did what I used to do and resorted to the internet to talk to people. I relied on people whom I only knew through social media to listen to the things I had to say, I expressed my feelings of anger, misery and frustration to people I had never even

met! That's what my life had come to, I couldn't even be myself to the people I loved but I was completely comfortable with sharing the fact I felt depressed, had cut my wrist or felt like dying to someone on the other end of a computer screen. I lived a lie, and it was the only way I felt I could live. I had spent the three previous years being hassled, bothered, questioned and examined for my actions and I was sick of it. It just wanted to be left alone so I could deal with it on my own.

Chapter 14 – A Life Changing Decision

Entering 2010 wasn't anything special to me. All I had achieved the previous year was smoking cannabis with friends regularly and not making a suicide attempt. I didn't feel proud of myself for anything, with the exception of a promotion to Bar Manager at the restaurant I had been working at the past few years. It wasn't much too brag about but at least it gave me a confidence boost from time to time. I had gotten myself into another relationship with a girl just before Christmas of the previous year as I wanted to give "love" another try. By now I had gotten over Stacy and the two of us were on really good speaking and friendship terms, plus she had a partner that I got on really well with. The new girl I got with wasn't anything like Stacy, or the girl from my previous relationship, and it was working out for the best. I felt genuinely loved, she was very interested in me and I felt content for the first time in a while. Suicide had faded to the furthest corners of my mind and even self-harm took a little break from time to time. Depression though was still showing up regularly though. The way in which I operated in the relationship was different to my previous efforts too. I didn't feel like trying taking the driving seat all the time, as that was a one of the factors as to why Stacy and I split up, and in fact my partner tried to most of the time, which I didn't mind it, for a while.

As the year went on I still felt the same monotonous feeling I had throughout 2009, the only difference was that I was in a longer relationship and that I had managed to keep most of my harmful thoughts at bay, which I didn't see as an achievement at the time. I knew I was still depressed but I had used weed and sex as a way of masking it this time round. In the latter half of that year I realised I wasn't happy and the relationship I was in didn't help the depression I had clouding me. Again, being the classy gentleman that I was called it off, at least this time I timed it better. I felt under the thumb in that relationship, plus my partner made some poor decisions, from my perspective, which made me question whether I needed that kind of negativity in my life. She had made a serious threat to one of my closest female friends which ended with her Dad coming down to my place of work and nearly punching me in the face over the bar that I managed on one quiet Sunday afternoon. That left me in tears. I didn't need a partner that was insecure over a friend of mine, I didn't need to be told what to do constantly and I didn't want to be tied down to someone who wasn't a positive influence. So I had to end it for my own peace of mind, which I desperately needed. As negative as my mind had been for the last five years I could still recognise that I didn't want any more of it around me if I could help it.

In the late summer of 2010 I was becoming massively reflective, way more than I had been throughout the peak of my depression. After five years of depression, anxiety, self-harm and suicide attempts I had a lot of experiences to think back over, which I did often. I wasn't in a relationship, nor was I looking for one, so I had a lot of time to myself during the day. I still worked at the same restaurant I had been at since late 2006, but I had also become the Kitchen Manager, and that kept me busy four evenings and two full days a week. For most work is dull but for me it was an escape from my mind. I genuinely enjoyed my job, mostly for the people I worked with and how much it challenged my skills. After work I always had my best friend Lewis, and sometimes Richard, around for a smoke and a video game or movie session. But it was the day time during the week that left me undistracted and paying attention to the depression. I found it incredibly difficult to stay motivated to do much more than listen to music, stare at the ceiling and over think my life, past and present. This went on more often than it should have but at least I had managed to minimalize the amount I self-harmed. Self-harm had become less of a habit and more of a reaction to a bad situation, unlike before where I was doing it regularly just to feel pain as often as I could. I remember, sadly, not having any weed one night and resorting to self-harm as I was feeling lower than dirt. In the earlier days of smoking cannabis I used it predominantly to help fight off my depressive thoughts and feelings, whilst still taking medication. I know, sad right? When you're that low you become prepared to do just about anything you can to yourself if it brings a happy feeling, even if it's a synthetic feeling and for a short while.

I was an emotional zombie during the day. I kept up my appointments with Mark most weeks just to let off some steam. I had been seeing him for nearly two years and I had got to the point where I felt like the sessions were only good for getting things off my chest rather than actually making progress with my life and helping me convert my mind set to something more positive. Although I had got my self-harm behaviours more under control than previous years I still had the urges almost every day. Mark was the only person I felt comfortable speaking with about this, I was still maintaining a positive image for the ones I loved. But I never shared with him that I had a suicidal contingency plan. Five years on I was still frustrated and depressed over my lack of ambition and purpose. "What am I supposed to do with my life?" This would usually be the first question I asked myself when in a depressive state in the day times and then I would follow up with, "I'm too much of a failure to do anything with my life." I had always believed that because I quit Sixth Form early and didn't make it to college or university to gain any qualifications that I was not educated enough to reach what I deemed to be a "success". When I looked at my Mum and Step Dad I saw success. They had a lovely home, nice cars, money and were both self-employed in careers that they were very passionate about. I believed that I could never reach that level. They had everything I wanted; happiness, success and were in love, as well as material possessions, and thinking of them brought me down. The image I had of them overshadowed my existence and made me look like the failure that I believed I was. I was ashamed of being who I was and the fact was doing nothing worthwhile with my time. As much as I loved being young, getting wrecked, playing video games and going to heavy metal gigs with friends I wanted something more, something real, something with purpose and the lack of it was beginning to send me into having strong suicidal thoughts again.

By the last quarter of 2010 I had managed to make more progress towards recovery than the previous four years combined. But it was inconsistent and I wasn't trying as hard as I could have. Like I mentioned, I kept self-harm to a minimum, cutting roughly once every few weeks, but the desires were getting stronger, along with my desire for suicide, due to the constant battle I had with the feeling of failure and a lack of purpose. It was eating me up daily but I spoke to no one about it because I was edging more towards committing suicide again and I knew that I would blow my cover if I spoke to anyone, other than Mark, about the fact I was still depressed. I had worked so hard to make my friends, family and work

colleagues believe that I was happy and I couldn't afford to start a snowball effect by starting off saying that I was low due to a lack of a life purpose. I would have my Mum, friends, etc. starting checking in on me every day making sure I wasn't cutting my wrists or storing up my pills. If I was going to make another attempt on my own life I have to do so without giving anything away.
One afternoon, in late 2010, I was all alone at my Nan's house, she had gone out for the day, and I was in a state of feeling low. I hadn't self-harmed in a few weeks but I was feeling the urge to. I kept thinking about when I could potentially kill myself. I envisioned myself falling asleep, after swallowing all my pills, and never waking up as I laid there on my bed. It was surprisingly warm in the conservatory where my bedroom was and I was beginning to sweat anxiously in my depressive state. This happened a lot when I fantasised, in a serious sense, about ending my life. As well as imagining myself dying I thought back to the worst events of my past, from cutting, to being bullied, to my break up with Stacy and to the overdose of 2008. When you're depressed and planning on killing yourself you think back to the worst experiences you've had because you want to convince yourself that your actions will be justified. "Why do I have to keeping feeling like this?" I asked myself lethargically. After staring at the ceiling for half an hour I decided to get off of my bed and take a shower. "This might make me feel a little better," I hoped. I walked to the bathroom with the same drooping shoulders like I always did when I was feeling down. I turned the taps on and looked at myself in the mirror for a few minutes whilst the water heated up. I stared blankly at myself whilst I kept on asking myself, "Why do I deserve this?" and, "Why do I have to keep putting up with this?" I hated feeling like this.

The shower had heated up and I stepped into the bath to let the hot water spray my face and cleanse the feeling of disappointment from my heart. When I felt depressed, in a non-frustrated or upset kind of way, I always had that expectation of my times in the shower. I really wanted the water to wash away my feelings but they never did. During this particular shower session I leant against the wall to my right whilst thinking, "I'm a failure and I want to die." My heart, face and the rest of my muscles were so limp I was just about holding myself up whilst I gazed into the splashing water around my feet. I looked down there for five minutes or so as the suicidal thoughts passed from one end of my mind to another. I wanted to cry but I couldn't, sometimes the depression was so heavy that I couldn't cry and instead the tears would stay compacted inside of me along with the emotions that they carried. The shower wasn't making me feel any better so I got out and made way to my room. What followed was when everything changed for me.

I dried myself off with my head hanging low. I put my underwear on and I noticed the mirror on the cupboard door at the end of my bed. I felt like looking at myself one last time; for whatever reason. I walked over to lock eyes with myself in the reflection. Just like I did in the bathroom I thought of suicide and in my head I was suggesting to myself that it was the right thing to do. But for the first time in *five years* another voice inside of me, which felt like it was coming from my soul, was saying things like, "C'mon Scott you're better than this," and, "You've got to keep fighting this shit. I hadn't experienced the fighting spirit within me for years and it felt quite alien. "You can do this Scott!" I could *hear* inside of me. I had no idea where this positive fighting talk was coming from but I started to feel good. With the encouragement I could hear within myself I started to consider living and fighting, which was then countered with thoughts like, "Dying would be better," and, "You're a failure Scott." I would then dip again for a moment. But then that would be countered with a voice saying, "No Scott, you're fucking awesome and you're a winner." Positive then negative, negative and then positive again. It was overwhelming and I could feel my chest tightening up. I wanted to be out of my skin and anywhere else. The battle inside of me between wanting to die and wanting to live was difficult to handle and make real sense of. I don't remember even remember looking at myself in the mirror after a while as all this inner conflict was causing me to zone out and disassociate.

The two sides inside my mind were battling it out to the death and I felt as if I was caught in the crossfire, like when I was present during the arguments between my Mum and Dad. After what seemed like a long time, but was probably only a minute, I couldn't take any more of this mental war so I snapped myself out of it. Then my mind went dead silent. The inner fight was no more and my mind was clear. Coming back to reality after being internalised so intensely was a weird transition that I can't describe effectively with words. It's more surreal than waking up from a deep sleep, it's more like waking up from an uncomfortable dream then being uncertain if it was real or not.
My next movements did feel more surreal than anything I had ever experienced in my whole life. They felt surreal because I didn't feel like I was the one in control of my own body.

My eyes slowly lifted from staring at the floor and in the reflection I could see myself once again, this time my eyes were locked with the ones staring back at me. Without consciously thinking I let my right hand tighten up with an extended index finger. My arm raised ninety degrees so that it was pointing at myself in the mirror. And that's when I said, in a very loud and affirmative tone; *"Scott, you're going to be HAPPY and you're going to MAKE SOMETHING OF YOUR LIFE!"*

What I had just commanded myself left me feeling shaken and slightly disorientated, it was almost like I had been possessed by some positive spirit that was motivating me to be happy. I had gone from barely breathing to breathing deeply in a matter of seconds whilst I consciously took in what had just happened to me. It was very surreal. I had no idea where those even came from but it felt right, it felt good. I couldn't remember the last time I motivated myself to do something so positive, let alone try and fight this urge to die. Normally I got over my urges to commit suicide, self-harm or feel depressed by distracting myself with things like video games, weed, seeing friends or music. But this was something completely different. I felt, for the first time in years, a true and genuine desire to live and to fight for a great life that I knew I deserved. As the adrenaline faded away and with my heart racing I walked back over to the bed to sit and continue comprehending what had just happened and what this really meant.

"What the *fuck* just happened?"

Chapter 15 – Recovery and Ascension

Shortly after sitting on bed in the heat of my Nan's conservatory I got up to get dressed and get something to eat. I did this on autopilot whilst I was internally focused and still trying to make sense of my "turning point". At the time I didn't see it as a turning point because I was still a little sceptical. I had tried to be more positive and pro-recovery a few times before and they always ended with me giving up and going back to square one so you can see why I would be sceptical at this point.
I had some many questions and ideas running through my head, at a pace that was usually carrying negative thoughts. But this time the questions and ideas were all positive, or at least positively curious. I could feel myself getting quite enthused over it actually. I was asking myself things

like, "What can I do to be more positive?", "How do I stop self-harming?", "How can I be a better person?". I had no answers for any of these questions but that didn't bother me. I believed in myself for the first time in over five years and I believed I would find answers to such questions, and, many more worthwhile questions that involved self-improvement.

I went to work that evening with a little more spring in my step. I felt genuinely happy to be going into work. I could feel a buzz in my chest and a broad smile on my face. It was rare for me to go into work this happy. I was effortlessly motivated, very unusual for me. Normally, if I wasn't high or in a good mood, I had to really psych myself up and sell myself the idea that work was going to go well. When I arrived into the kitchen to start my shift I threw myself into my role. I went at it with great enthusiasm and effort. I was being as observant as I could to make sure I was on top of carrying out my job. I made my awareness stay on high alert so that I could be proactive as well as reactive. I wanted to do an amazing job and I wanted people to notice the shift in me. Being recognised and acknowledged by people had always been something I craved and in my attempt at a genuine turn around I wanted people to notice. In the past five years of my struggles with mental health I had rarely, if at all, felt proud of myself. Although I was only about six hours into trying sort my life out and improve myself I did feel proud. I used this positive emotion to keep up the momentum at work. Rather than watch the clock I kept striving to be on top of my game as an employee.
Before I knew it the shift was over and we all finished on a high note. It had been a steady shift but combining my enthusiasm with that of my colleagues we got through it successfully and could walk away feeling good. I felt especially positive. I had a good feeling about my recovery. I felt confident and optimistic that things were gonna be OK. It's amazing how shouting at myself in front of a mirror could help give me the motivation I needed.

Between that surreal moment of standing in front of my bedroom mirror, and my strong inner voice breaking free of it's negative ties, and the end of 2010 I spent the majority of my time trying to get my mind to produce positive thoughts. I can assure you that I was not an easy task. The test really began on the second day of recovery. I remember waking up the way I usually did, with my head thinking, "Oh fuck sake, I can't be bothered with life." But once I had got up and walked to the kitchen to make myself a coffee I remembered what happened the day before. By reliving that turning point in my head as I sipped my hot cup of coffee I knew that I could not let myself slip into my habits of letting myself be easily defeated by my emotions before that day had even begun. I said to myself silently that this was going to be another day that I live with a positive attitude; "It's going to be a good day."

I went through this routine almost every day for the rest of the year. "It's going to be alright.", "I'm going to be as positive as I can be." and "I'm going to do a great job." were all phrases I would say to myself in the morning as I woke up. Waking up and feeling good was hard to begin with. I spent the last five years waking up and not wanting to do so. Changing habits that you have been engaging in for a long time are difficult to change regardless of what they are and this was the mother of all challenges from my perspective. But it did get easier as time went on. Of course, there were days where I really struggled to motivate myself no matter how hard I tried. And just because I could mould a positive mindset in the morning it didn't mean that I could stay that way for the whole day. During this time I did relapse and end up cutting myself from time to time but it didn't have the same effect during or afterwards. What I mean by this is that during the cutting I wouldn't be as aggressive towards myself, or cut as much as I used to, and afterwards I wouldn't be half as disappointed with myself like I did over the past few years. In fact I didn't even feel like it would give me the same sense of "calmness" that it used to. I didn't feel like I had gone back to the start of my recovery journey each time I put a blade to my skin. Instead I could say to myself, "OK, this has happened but I've got to keep trying."

With each day passing I found myself trying to tackle my emotions and thoughts at earlier stages when facing my triggers. Anything from working being stressful, feeling lonely, being criticised or not knowing what to do with my life were all triggers that I seemed to encounter on a daily basis. This meant that my recovery journey was being apprehended regularly, which also meant I had to hold myself together and not get brought down by such circumstances or perspectives. As I said before, it wasn't easy. But as challenging situations arose in my head I would give myself some verbal encouragement or "wisdom" sooner rather than later. I found this to be more effective than to dwell upon it and deal with it later. If I didn't give myself some positive reinforcement early on then the negativity would play on my mind and I would fail in preventing to feel the need to self-harm. When things did go wrong I would try to say to myself, "It doesn't matter.", "I'm better than this.", or I would push myself to find a way to fix the problem. One time I had finished work in the kitchen and I went to the bar to have a drink. I wore black skinny jeans, a black t-shirt with a gruesome design on it bearing the band name Carnifex and a black snap back hat. A gentleman in his early thirties stood next to where I ordered a cider from my colleague behind the bar. The guy looked me up and down and said sarcasticly, "You look colourful."

If you had or have problems with depression and anxiety how would that make you feel? Quite uneasy to say the least I'm sure. If this had happened to me a year or two before hand I would have felt very uncomfortable and it probably would have played on my mind for the rest of the evening until I got home and cut myself. But this was another opportunity to think about how I *should* respond rather than how I *could* respond. I held my composure for a second and looked the man in the eye and smiled then continued to talk to my colleague at the bar. I felt pretty good for not getting angry or upset and that was the situation dealt with. I forgot about it by the time I had taken a few sips of my pint. For most people this is an illustration of a moment that is easy to control, but for someone who is trying to overcome years of depression and anxiety this can be a difficult task.

A little further down the line of that year I was met with, quite literally, a heated moment. On a busy Saturday night whilst working in the kitchen I was handed a salad from one of the waitresses. At this time the kitchen was hot, noisy and had a combination of ten chefs and the front of house team members running around trying to do their best. As the salad was passed to me the waitress said something in relation to why the meal had come back. Over the noise of the equipment, music and shouting staff I couldn't make out exactly what she had said to me so, like any normal person would, I asked her, in a very calm voice, to repeat what she had said. I didn't get the co-operative response I was expecting. "JUST GIVE ME THE FUCKING SALAD!" she screamed. The whole back of house area went silent. If the music hadn't been on our speaker system playing you could have heard a pin drop. But how did I react? Even as a strong minded person how would you want to react? Lash back with profanity? Walk away and cry? I'm sure there would be many more negative reactions an individual could carry out rather than positive ones. Thanks to my extensive efforts to control my thoughts and emotions over the last couple of months I was able to make the best possible move I could comprehend at the time. In a soft and calm tone I simply said, "Sorry I didn't hear what you asked me?" I could have said something of a nasty nature to her like, "Don't fucking talk to me like that!" Or I could have let it bring me down, dwell upon it and let it impair my thinking, which would have messed up the flow of service as I was the one in control of communicating all the food orders. This person had also taken the piss out of me in a meeting a few years before hand when I overheard her talking about me saying that she thought I was going to cry when she asked me to do something. But no, I responded in a more than justified way. I felt so proud of myself for being the bigger and better person in that situation. Plus I got the satisfaction of her embarrassing herself for her childlike attitude.

My efforts to better myself and be more positive didn't go unnoticed at work. I was given the kitchen manager position, more responsibilities and better pay because I had proved I could handle the pressure and I demonstrated good leadership skills. I had to take that position whilst also being the bar manager. That's not something I could have done earlier in the year. Being rewarded for my worth ethic was a big achievement for me because I now had a tangible result for overcoming my mental health challenges. I didn't need people to recognise me for turning my self around but it made a big difference to my confidence and my ego. If you're an employer please make time to recognise your team for the work they put it. A face to face conversation is the best place to start. Even without struggling with mental health everyone likes to be recognised for the things that they do, even if they do it every day and it's their job role. A well done and a thank you go a long way, especially if someone is mentally suffering and they feel worthless. By recognising their efforts you could be put a smile on their face, give them self-confidence or even save their lives. Think about that for a moment.

By the end of 2010 I had achieved a lot more emotional control and I was more at peace with myself. I was practically a new person. Negative experiences were getting fewer and fewer and when they did come at me I was mentally prepared for anything that tried to stop me or slow me down. I began to welcome negative circumstances because I wanted to gain some experience and strengthen my mind. I got a sense of fun out of it. Anything that came to me was either denied a chance of affecting me or was used as a way to better myself. I could take a moment and change

it according to my desires if I tried hard enough and if it was worth me doing so.
I truly felt I had beat depression, anxiety and self-harm. It had been a while since I cut and it felt so good coming to the end of the year on a high note. I can't describe what that freedom felt like, I can only imagine it carried the same sensation as a person leaving prison after living a long sentence for a crime they didn't commit. If you have ever seen The Shawshank Redemption you will know what I mean. I had also become confident enough to have my scars on show. I wasn't ashamed of what I had done to my body. Just like everyone else on the planet I was, and always will be, a human being with emotions and obstacles to overcome. I had developed a carefree attitude towards having my scars out and the beautiful thing was that no one asked me about them and as far as I could tell barely anyone even noticed. I wasn't getting funny looks or any harassment in public or amongst my piers. Being able to just go out and enjoy my life was a feeling that I had been craving for years. I was more outgoing, I even danced in our local club (if I was a little drunk), and I began to say yes to people's invitations to come round their house, parties and raves. These were not things I was usually comfortable with. The freedom I now had from mental health problems gave me a new lease on life and it was fabulous.

Going into 2011 I was more optimistic than I had been my whole life. I remember saying to myself at the beginning of the year that this would be *my year*. I wanted to climb the ranks in my job at the restaurant, I wanted to have fun with my friends and I wanted to spend time with my family. From time to time I stood in front of the mirror in my bedroom, the same mirror I stood in front of and demanded happiness and success from myself. I recognised that moment as my turning point so I didn't see any harm in using that method as a way to encourage myself.
I was already doing well in my job and having fun with friends so I just needed to keep that up but I needed to invest in time with my family. You have already read into my past through the earlier chapters in this book and it's no secret that I had rocky relationships with my Dad and Step Dad, as well as my Mum from time to time. I practised cultivating people at work, both staff and customers, by demonstrating a positive attitude and being flexible to people's personalities. I used these tactics to build better relationships with my Dad and Step Dad, because they were the two people I felt I had disappointed through my behaviours. Despite our arguments, disagreements and lack of understanding I still looked up to

them and all I wanted was for us to get along. No, not just get along, I wanted us to have a deep sense of love for each other which would be illustrated in our behaviours towards one another. That's how I wanted my whole family to be and I wanted to be a part of that.

In the few years I had lived at my Nan's house I had declared myself the black sheep of the family. Being distant from the rest of my family during my depressed years was my choice because I believed it to be easier than getting into arguments or feeling uncomfortable all the time. But this was a "new year new me" kind of thing and I knew it was time to change this, and it was down to me. In fact, looking back it was the last thing I needed to do in order to claim the title of "fully recovered". It had been a few months since I last self-harmed and even though I felt free of my struggles the urges still popped up now and again. I suppose it was like a withdrawal symptom. The only area in my life I was not 100% satisfied with was the relationship between me and my close family. Perhaps sorting that out would kill off the remaining self-harm urges I had and enable me to be even more positive.
So, I made it my mission to rebuild my relationship with my family, mainly with my Dad and Step Dad. I knew this would take time but I had to start somewhere by giving a little; something I should have done a long time ago. I got into the habit of texting and calling them out of the blue and I arranged to see them more than I used to. Like the other people I had cultivated in my life I would try to put their interests before my own with simple things like asking them how they were doing, taking an interest in the things that they were doing and offering to help them if they needed me for something. I'm confident my family could see a positive change in me and they could see I wanted to be a part of the family, both and my Dad's and Mum's side, because everything between us just got smoother and smoother. We were more respectful, more giving and more loving towards one another. I could go round my Mum's or Dad's house and feel completely comfortable instead of feeling anxious, distant and judged. Improving my relationship with all my parents was my second greatest achievement yet, after that of taking control of my self-destructive habits.

The rest of 2011 went exactly as I planned it, and more. In fact 2011 opened more doors for me than I thought was possible for a person of twenty years of age. In the first few months of 2011 I had almost forgotten about my past and the five year struggle. I didn't want to think about it. Not because it bothered me, but because I had no time for

negativity any more. I still worked six days a week in the same restaurant I had been at for nearly five years and it was going really well. I was a well respected senior member of staff and I was proud of myself. I was single, but that was my choice. I had been in relationships for the majority of the past six years and I wanted a break and just to stay focused on myself. Most of my relationships ended badly so I stayed away from them. I felt loved by my family and friends, which I had plenty of, so what did I have to feel negative about? Nothing at all and I felt FUCKING AMAZING. Pardon my language.
But they weren't the only blessings that life was prepared to hand me. My whole world was about to unfold from this new beginning. I arrived for work one Friday and my boss Jo was in the office. She seemed to be in a good mood, she generally was anyway, but Friday could be hit or miss as it was usually the day where she had lots of admin work to do and her boss sometimes had a shitty phone conversation with her. After our general chit chat about the business and how we were doing in our personal lives she asked me if I had ever heard of "The Secret". I was both sceptical and intrigued. I asked what it was all about as "The Secret" could have meant anything. She suggested I go and watch it, or read the book. As soon as I finished my morning shift I went home and downloaded it straight away. I watched it with an open mind, just as Jo suggested I do. Now, I have always been open minded on things that were "outside the ordinary" and with my new found outlook on life I decided to give the teachings in this film a go. The people in the video had very convincing stories and the quotations from famous people that were shared in the film were very inspiring for me. If you have not seen or read The Secret I highly recommend it, but, only when you're ready to receive it. If I had seen this film during my years of depression I would have written it off straight away. I highly recommend that you wait till you're in a more stable place before reading or watching it too as it does require an open mind and because it's such a positive film and book it may be too much for you if you're in a bad place right now.

Anyway I followed and applied it's teachings for a month and came to the conclusion that this was going to be something I would continue to follow for the rest of my life. For me it was enlightening and empowering. Not only had I gone from negative to positive in the past six months I now left like I was beginning to live an enhanced life through these teachings. Of course some of my friends and family thought I was just following some ridiculous positive thinking book but for me it was way more than that. It worked for me and that's all that mattered. And that's all that should matter for you. If you find a book, programme, philosophy, religion, etc. works for you by helping you think better thoughts and take better actions then stick to it no matter what everyone else around you says. What doesn't work for them might work for you and vice versa. I don't want to reveal the teachings of "The Secret" as I may spoil and undersell it but I will say that watching the film, and then reading the book, did set me up to start a journey that I never imagined I could go on. I was more positively charged than ever. I wanted to figure out what I could now do with my life and I was hungry for knowledge that would influence me to succeed in life. I was beginning to develop a success mindset. Imagine that; me, after all the things I had been through, now creating a successful mindset for myself. The contrast between how positive I had become versus how negative I was only a year before was insanely opposite. I had never seen anyone change that much before, not anyone I knew anyway. Up until late 2011 I spent the majority of my time doing about three things. One; Applying the teachings from The Secret and other motivational books in that genre. I was beginning to build a small library of success books! Two; Working my ass off to be the best I could be in my job. I earned a promotion to Assistant Manager too! Three; I was having spending lots of time having fun with my friends and family. It was beautiful. I had become the social person I had always wanted to be. I was confident, fun and interesting around people. Being asked to go out with people for drinks or get togethers was pretty exciting and being wanted by people was important to me. I have always had attachment issues so having people want my company because they liked who I was just made me feel important. Who doesn't want to feel important anyway?

One thing I never mentioned previously was that in early 2009 Stacy and I had managed to rekindle our friendship. Yes, that was going on in the background of all this. Things were good between us on the whole. She was seeing a guy for a while, whom I befriended actually. The three of us, sometimes accompanied by Lewis, used to hang out quite regularly. Anyway back to 2011 (there is a point to this!), around August Stacy and her partner broke up. Stacy and I had always been close, apart from when we broke up obviously, and I was starting to fall for her again. Of course I valued our friendship and I didn't want to ruin that, especially with what I had been through with her already. Though I did let the cat out of the bag on her birthday that year. Lewis held a party at his place and it fell on Stacy's birthday so us lot and a load of friends went to his for drinks,

music and lots of banter. Without a doubt I got very drunk and stoned. Lewis said that Stacy and I could sleep in his bed, which we were both cool with. We were way passed any awkward feelings of the past; we weren't kids any more and we were very open minded. Before we fell asleep I said to Stacy, in my wasted state, "I still love you." I then laid on the bed and fell asleep instantly.
The next morning I woke up and didn't remember how the previous night ended, not straight away at least. When I did remember what I had confessed to Stacy I stayed quiet about it hoping that it would never be brought up again. Fortunately for me it wasn't brought up again.
But in October that year it was brought up, completely out of the blue, and, I was driving her about so I couldn't even make an excuse to escape. Whilst driving about in Maidstone Stacy asked me what I meant that night at Lewis's party. Before I could answer I got an exciting feeling that perhaps we could get back together. I had learned to be optimistic and I had drastically bettered myself since we broke up three years ago. I had a good feeling about it. All I had to do was be honest and tell her how I really felt. I told her, "I meant what I said, I love you still and I don't think I ever stopped loving you since we have been split up." At this point I thought I had potentially sealed the deal. No. The response I got wasn't what I had hoped for. She explained to me that she didn't want to ruin our friendship. Being in the friend zone was cool before hand, but since confessing my true feelings I struggled to suppress them any longer. I didn't say much back to her, in fact I was pretty silent and feeling very disappointed. She could sense it and tried to comfort me. Eventually I managed to get out of a child-like sulking state and carry on appreciating the close friendship that we had.

Before 2011 came to a close I could look back and confirm to myself that this was the year I had taken full control of my mental health and my life. As well as the job promotion there was another big blessing coming my way. In December I went to hang out with Stacy like I often did. I sat on her bed and started engaging in conversation with her. She seemed more happier and smiley than usual. I started to get butterflies in my stomach for some reason too. I couldn't figure out why I was feeling so excited and anxious. And that's when she said, "I think you and me should try again." If it's not obvious, that meant she wanted us to try a relationship again. I remember being absolutely stunned at the time. I didn't expect Stacy to suggest this, baring in mind only two months ago she had said that she didn't want to ruin our friendship. My heart was racing with excitement but my head was telling me to sleep on it. And with that I responded with, "Give me a bit of time to think about it." To be honest I knew at this point I was going to say yes to her. In fact I gave it no thought and the next day we were back together again. Boy was I over the moon and in love again!

Chapter 16 – A Happy Ending and Life Lessons

In the beginning of 2012 I had been clean of self-harm for over a year. As you can imagine I was so pleased to be able to deal with negativity without resorting to self-destruction. I had, and still have plenty of scars on my body but that didn't bother me. I could look at them without feeling ashamed and instead I could remind myself of how far I've come. Things between Stacy and I were also spectacular. In May we had moved into our first place together and our apartment was beautiful. Just before we moved in I was offered a job by a customer whilst serving them in the bar of the restaurant I worked at. The hotel chain that I moved to was a bigger and better company and my salary increased by about five thousand pounds. I was offered the job because I gave this woman and her colleagues great service. That in itself was an interesting story. Whilst managing a shift on a quiet Monday night I had sent the person working on the bar home to save on staff spending. The restaurant staff had also finished about half an hour before hand. The bar was due to close at eleven and at half ten we had no customers in the building. I was also fifty pounds away from achieving our sales target for the day. I stood behind the bar waiting for time to pass so I could close up and go home. I looked out the window and there was nobody in sight. Our front door was open, the bright neon lights that formed our restaurants name was highly visible in the dark and music was playing through the speakers located inside and outside the business. I really wanted to achieve our sales target but with no-one lurking around outside it didn't look like I'd be serving any more drinks that night. Through what I had learnt in The Secret I stood there and visualised a group of people walking through the door and coming to me to spend fifty pounds. Quarter to eleven came and still nobody. Ten to eleven came and still no one. I thought to myself, "Nobody is coming." But something inside me was saying, "wait!" I hesitantly walked a few steps towards the front door and out of nowhere a group of about five people walked through the door. I welcomed them with a huge smile on my face and quickly turned around to get into action. Some beers and cocktails were ordered but it didn't quite come to fifty pounds, it was just over thirty pounds. I wasn't phased by this because I was over the moon that I had imagined this happening and then it actually happened. Before she could start her drink a woman from the group came over to me and asked me what my position was. I explained to her that I was the assistant manager and that I had plenty of experiences in all areas of the restaurant. Her response was, "I was really impressed with the way you served us, we are always looking for people like you to work in our business. Here's my email address, send me your CV and I will arrange to have a chat with you." At that moment I could feel my stomach doing back flips, my hands shaking and my heart beating really fast. I had been looking for a new job for about a month at this point and I couldn't believe this opportunity had landed on me. To cut a long story short I went for an interview and got a job as an assistant food and beverage manager within a large hotel.

This was the first time I had really paid attention to my instincts and not the logical part of my brain in order to manifest a great blessing. This experience taught me to be very alert if I could "sense something" without having any logic or facts to go on as it meant something significant was about to happen to me. I got the same feeling a few weeks later when Stacy and I were buying our first home. We had been through many painstaking tasks to get ourselves on the property ladder and when we were driving about one day I got a strong feeling inside of me that I had felt only once before; moments before I was offered a new job. When we got home we received a call telling us that the apartment we had been trying to buy was now officially ours. My life was positively expanding so fast I couldn't believe how much "luck" I was having. In October 2012 I got a promotion to be a food and beverage manager for a new hotel that was due to open early 2013, which meant another pay rise and more responsibilities. And before 2012 came to a close Stacy fell pregnant with our first baby! What a journey life had become! Rather than bore you with every detail I want to skip ahead now to the middle of 2017, roughly about the time when I started to write this book. In that time Stacy and I had, and still have, two wonderful daughters, I got another promotion, my salary had increased by eleven thousand pounds (versus what I was earning early 2012) and I had also come to the realisation that my life purpose was to help young people with struggle self-harm and mental health problems.

The idea of the previous paragraphs are not to make anyone jealous or for me to boast about the things I had achieved by the age of twenty seven. I want to illustrate what can be achieved even when you're facing problems with your mental health. They say that when you hit rock bottom the only way you can go is up. I hope the experiences I've shared with you in this book prove the facts in this old saying. I'm also a strong believer in everything happening for a reason. Napoleon Hill, author of *Think and Grow Rich*, said that "Every adversity carries with it the seed of an equivalent benefit." I strongly believe that I went through my battles with mental health so that I would be lead to finding my purpose in life. I know to some close minded people that may sound ridiculous, but you're not a close minded reader are you? I thought not. My purpose, or life goal, or whatever you wish to call it, is to motivate, inspire and empower young people that self-harm to live more positively and to follow their dreams. At the age of twenty two I demanded of myself to find out what my life was all about. I had always been curious of unanswered questions and there's nothing more important than knowing one's purpose in life. But it wasn't till about the age of twenty four did I realise that wanted to help people, mostly the young, that self-harm and suffer with depression, anxiety, etc.

Two years to figure out my definite goal may seem long but honestly one of the biggest lessons I learnt in happiness and mental stability is that being in pursuit of some sort of goal, aim or purpose is one of the best ways in wanting to stay alive. Goals, no matter how large or small, are powerful and positive motivators. The brain releases dopamine when forming goals, taking action towards goals and even more when you actually achieve them. If you have heard of dopamine before you may know that it makes you feel good. Good enough to make you satisfied and change you from a negative to a positive frame of mind. You may already know what your purpose or life goal is, or, you may not. And yet you may kind of *think* you know what it is. None of these are particularly bad but from what I've experienced I truly believe that having a purpose in life can make the difference between wanting to live a wonderful life and wanting to end it all. I think that everyone has a purpose to be found or a life goal to achieve. Do you know yours? Have you been searching for it? If you already know what it is that you're doing with your life then that's great, you're already one of the few people that are becoming successful and living the life that they want. But if you haven't discovered or decided what you want to do with your time on this planet then I please beg of you to figure this out. You can be or do anything you want when you put your mind to it and take appropriate action. If you need some outside motivation just Google "inspirational quotes" or something of that nature. The internet can actually be good sometimes. It's filled with positive quotations from successful and inspiring people. As much as I'm placing emphasis on the importance of knowing what to do with your life please don't stress over this and think that it all needs to be figured out right away. I didn't understand what my purpose was till I was twenty four. It took me two years to figure out what I really wanted to do. It took me four years to go from knowing what I wanted to do to actually achieving a tangible result; publishing this book and getting it into the hands of those whom could benefit from it. Everyone is different. Some discover it from an early age as to what they're passionate about and some take years. Don't be put off by this. At the end of the day we all have the greatest resource of them all; time. If you just put in a little time each day into sitting down and brainstorming or talking with someone who is supportive and knows you well then you'll figure it out sooner rather than later. Think about what you're passionate about and what you're good at. This is the ideal starting point, especially that part about passion.

It may take a while but it will be so worth it. Since being in pursuit of my definite purpose I have been satisfied in the fact that I know what direction my life is heading. It may take ten years or more for you to discover and achieve your life goal, it may not. Time is always going to pass and you will be much happier spending a life time in pursuit of a dream than you would just merely existing, studying subjects without knowing why, doing a job that you hate, scraping by with little money and living without meaning. You were destined for great things, you deserve them. One last thing about the pursuit of your goals and dreams is that life has a really weird way of letting you discovering things that are worth while. Life loves to throw you off or lead you down strange paths that seem unnecessary and unpleasant but it will give you answers and what you want in the end if you just have a little faith in yourself. I probably wouldn't have a purpose as meaningful as the one I have if I didn't suffer with depression, anxiety and self-harm. In a strange way I'm grateful for my struggles because I have used them to shape the life I want to live. And because of this, if I was to live my life over again I would do most of the same way. I'm ashamed of some of the mistakes I've made but I'm not ashamed of my mental health.

This brings me on to another important lesson I have learnt through my struggles. Shame is a choice, not a permanent result. This may be hard to accept but it's true. I am not ashamed of my mental health problems, the fact I have self-harmed or the scars on my body. It wasn't easy for me think like this at the time but now I can, and so can you. Shame can often come as a result of how other people make you feel. When that happens it's easy to accept what they say or do and then you begin to feel ashamed of yourself. Other people make it easy to upset vulnerable individuals. I had plenty of occasions at home where my self-harming behaviours would make my family ask me, "How do you think this makes us feel?" Every time I was asked something like that it would make me feel guilty and ashamed of myself for hurting them. But that was my choice at the time. Don't get me wrong I never wanted to upset anyone that I cared about but due to my health my urges to hurt myself were far greater than my desires to care for myself. That's nothing to be ashamed of. I don't need to be ashamed just because my mental health wasn't as good as it could be. You don't need to be ashamed of your mental health or your self-harm scars. Mental health has had it's stigma but it's becoming better understood by more and more people everyday. One of the key ways to put an end to the stigma is for more and more people to stop feeling ashamed of their mental health, scars, etc. and instead to accept their health and feel more comfortable with it. You're going to feel better about your mental health by accepting it. Choosing to accept your condition really is the key to not feeling ashamed. It's very similar to accepting your sexual orientation. When I started to have sexual urges towards men, as well as women, I had a portion of shame in me. That was until I fully accepted it and began to open up to my friends and family about it. The more you can accept it the more others around you will accept it. Other people might not get it but they will learn to accept it. From acceptance you will find it easier to talk about. Talking about it is another key to not feeling ashamed of your mental health, self harm scars, etc.

Ah, talking about it, I guess there people reading this book who have already been told, "you've got to be open and talk about your problems." Am I right? Talking and mental health seem to go hand in hand. Without a doubt talking about your feelings, thoughts or mental health is without a shadow of a doubt the single most important ingredient for recovery, or, living a better life alongside mental health difficulties. Talking, or rather communication as a whole, is one of the most important aspects of human relationships full stop, not just in mental well-being. Over the many years of human existence we have learned to communicate to one other in order to live more comfortably, succeed and survive. Without communication we would all perish. I know that may seem dramatic but it's true. Imagine if we all kept our mouths closed or never wrote messages to each other. What would that look like? How would you behave if everyone around you didn't say a word? How would you feel? Would you trust anyone? Would you know what their intentions were? Would you have any idea as to what they were thinking? No. You'd have to wait for them to act and by then any potential harm has already been done. When the damage has been done it's pretty hard to reverse. The exact same rule applies to you. How would your friends feel if you never spoke to them about your struggles and you self-harmed? How would your family feel if you never verbalised your emotional difficulties and committed suicide? What could anyone do at that point? I feel that I need to make these extreme illustrations to signify the importance of "opening up". I know for one that opening up about your negative thoughts and feelings isn't easy at all, especially to those whom you care about. Like me you probably don't want to bother, upset or hurt them. Telling your parents that you self-harm isn't easy. Telling your friends that you feel depressed isn't easy. Telling a therapist that you feel suicidal isn't easy. But do you know what's harder than all of those things? Living a life where you feel all alone with your problems. Feeling alone in your battles with mental health, or any form of challenge that life throws at you, is such a miserable experience. I can say that hand on heart that when I didn't open up and have someone to talk to when I felt so low it just made me feel even worse. Being alone, having to hide cuts and bottling up my emotions was like being a ghost. I would watch the world go by and feel like everyone else had everything going for them whilst I suffered and no one would even notice. Please, talk. Talk to someone. A friend, a relative or even a stranger on a call line. Our emotions were not designed to be silenced. They were designed to be expressed. Your emotions will seek expression sooner or later. Wouldn't you rather let out that negativity constructively instead of letting the pressure build up and explode in an uncontrollable way? I hope so because I want you to enjoy your life. I want you to be able to open up when shit hits the fan. I want you to live with and even overcome mental illness where it's possible, not suffer from it.

If you can't talk to someone close to you like a friend or relative you need to find someone ASAP. Maybe a teacher? Perhaps a work colleague?

There are plenty of phone-lines, that are free, that you can call. The people on the other end are their to listen and will not judge. Believe it or not sometimes that's all you need; someone to listen to the things you've got going on inside your mind. Your doctor is certainly someone you should be talking to if you're feeling depressed, anxious, self-harming or have suicidal intentions. They can point you in the right direction and get you a referral to local mental health services. I know it feels weird talking about your unpleasant thoughts to people but it will get easier to do the more you do it. But you've got to start opening that mouth of yours and let people know that you need help! There's no shame in that. We all need help from time to time and some people just need more help than others. It's a fact of life and no good person will judge you for needing help. In fact they will respect you and probably feel motivated to put a smile back on your face.

There's one last thing I'd like to say now and this is directed at those who don't understand mental health problems and to those who have a person in their life, perhaps a friend or family member, that is having difficulties with mental health. You cannot allow yourself to judge them in any way, shape or form. You can't get angry with them because of their problems. You must do your absolute best to remain calm, caring and patient. You may have had similar experiences and you might have a slight understanding but if you're displaying your frustrations and having a go at them then you're only damaging them, no matter what words you use. In my experiences, and in the experiences of many people I have spoken to, it's very easy for parents and friends to say or do things that have a negative effect on someone who is mentally struggling even though they "just want to help". You can't raise your voice at your child because you have noticed cuts on their arm. You can't call your friend boring because they're too anxious to come outside. You can't call your teenager lazy because their too depressed to climb out of bed. Any form of communication that lacks empathy really isn't helping. As you may already know people pick up more from your tone when talking than your actual words. People forget this all the time when trying to "help" someone who is struggling with depression, anxiety, etc. I'm confident that you really want to help your son, daughter, friend, student, etc. but if you're talking in a way that sounds aggressive, condescending, frustrated, disappointed or even sarcastic then you're doing more harm than good. I know you care about them and want to help them but you've got to talk to them in a way that is very gentle, calm and soothing. Otherwise they

will NOT let you in. That's the last thing you want isn't it? As soon as you raise your voice or act disappointed they will become defensive. It's human nature to do so when we feel attacked. They may not outwardly express that defence but inside they shut you off, or worse they could soak up your frustrations and start blaming themselves for their mental health. That's far worse in my experience.
I *highly* suggest that you let them know that you're there for them and that you make sure your actions back up those words. We've all had someone make us feel like their available in the time of need but never deliver on that promise. You can't afford to do that if you really care about them. They need as much support as they can get and you need to be one of the people they can count on to support them. Don't let them feel like they need to do this all on their own. Remind them that it's okay to have someone help them. Unless they're showing signs of damaging behaviour don't force them to into getting help. Some people take longer to get through to than others so don't over probe them with questions, I know you want answers but if you want them to open up you must be patient and just start by letting them know that you're there for them. I didn't find it easy at first opening up to anyone in my family but my Mum eventually did a good job in making herself available to me without hassling me for answers. As time went on I felt that I could come to her with my problems and I could answer her questions. I know everyone is different but in order to help some one you've got to be prepared to wait for them to come to you. They will come to you as long as you demonstrate your ability to be approachable.

If you have just discovered a loved one, a friend, student, etc. has self-harmed or is struggling mental you need to approach them with open arms and a gentle voice. You must also be prepared for them to close you off. I can tell you now that this will happen quite often in the beginning, and perhaps longer. If you want answers and feel that you need more of an insight than what my story has offered then I suggest you go online and look at some websites that have authority to give information about depression, self-harm and other mental health related topics. Again, talking to your doctor is a good idea.
Once again please don't get angry with someone because they have self-harmed, tried to take their own life, are feeling depressed etc. because you're going to keep making them want to hurt themselves or at least feel like absolute shit. I'm not saying that you're not entitled as a parent, friend or whatever to feel frustrated because you are. All you want to do

is help them and when they shut you off or keep doing the same damaging behaviours it really is frustrating. But you have got to let that frustration out elsewhere. If your daughter is frustrating you because she doesn't seem to listen to your positive suggestions then you should speak to your partner about it, or a friend or even a counsellor. You need someone to talk to as well. Give it time, be approachable, be a good listener and they will eventually come to you.

I can honestly say that writing this book has be a roller-coaster of emotions for me but now that it has come to an end I feel proud of myself. For whatever reason you're reading this book, whether it's to feel like you're not alone, read a personal story or gain an insight I want to say I'm proud of you. I can imagine that you the reader have good intentions because you wanted to gain something from reading this and to be able to use whatever it is that you've gained from this book to better someone's life; yours or someone else's. That's something to be proud. Finally, don't let your mind or emotions get the better of you or someone close to you. Care and communicate. If you're really struggling you've got to reach out and ask for help, there's no other way. And if you can sense that someone is really struggling be bold and do everything in your power to be the one who gives a helping hand. The road to recovery isn't short, straight or smooth but when everyone comes together great things can be achieved. No one can do this on their own and that's perfectly fine.

Thank you.

Post Script

November 2017, I relapsed.

To be continued...